Dr. Denmark Said It!

Advice to Mothers from America's Most Experienced Pediatrician

Madia Linton Bowman

Dr. Denmark Said It!
Madia L. Bowman
ISBN: 978-0-9703814-1-5

First published, 1998.
Second revised edition, 2001.
Third revised edition, 2004.
Fourth revised edition 2006.
Fifth revised edition, 2015.

Cover design by Steven Bowman

Printed in the United States of America.

Disclaimer

The ideas, procedures, and suggestions in this book are intended to supplement, not replace, the medical advice of a trained professional. All matters regarding your health require medical supervision. Consult your physician before adopting the suggestions in this book, as well as concerning any condition that may require diagnosis or medical attention. The author disclaims any liability arising directly, or indirectly, from the use of this book.

In loving memory of my treasured mentor and friend,
Dr. Leila Alice Daughtry Denmark.

Schedules..32

Naptime..34

Five Months..34

Food, Schedules, Sleep..34

Weaning..37

Sleep..37

Two Years..39

Food, Schedules, Sleep..39

Sleep Disturbances..40

Baby Schedule Summary..42

Immunizations..43

Chapter 2: Danger Signs Indicating Emergency........................47

Fever..47

Abdominal Pain..48

Other Signs of Emergency..49

Chapter 3: Common Ailments..51

Stomachache..51

Motion Sickness..53

Headaches..53

Skin..54

Cuts..54

Scrapes and Scratches..54

Severe Infection..55

Burns..56

Eczema..57

Rashes (General)..58

Poison Ivy or Poison Oak..58

Athlete's Foot..60

Ringworm..60

Impetigo..60

Sunburn..61

Boils..61

Chapped Skin..62

Blisters (friction)..62

Bites and Stings..63

Bee, Wasp, Fire Ant..63

Ticks..63

Table of Contents

Foreword..i

Acknowledgments..iii

Introduction...vii

Photos...ix

Chapter 1: Care of Infants...1

Newborn...4

Schedules..4

Crying Infant...6

Feeding...8

Breastfeeding..8

Premature Infant...9

Supplements...10

Spitting Up...12

Colic...13

Weight Gains...15

Postpartum...15

Positioning the Infant...16

Furniture Use...19

Quietness...20

Sunshine...20

Jaundice..21

Pacifiers and Thrush..21

Bathing...23

Clothing..24

Feet and Shoes...26

Diaper Rash..27

Teething..28

Three Months..28

Schedules..28

Homemade Baby Food..31

Four Months..32

Older women likewise are to be reverent in their behavior, not malicious gossips, nor enslaved to much wine, teaching what is good, that they may encourage the young women to love their husbands, to love their children, to be sensible, pure, workers at home, kind, being subject to their own husbands, that the word of God may not be dishonored.

—Titus 2:3-5

Mosquito and Other Common Insect Bites..............................64
Minor Dog and Cat Bites..............................64
Venomous Snake Bites..............................64
Lice..............................65
Swallowing Objects..............................65
Blow to the Head..............................65
Conjunctivitis..............................66
Fainting..............................67
Menstrual Pain..............................67
Minor Mouth Sores..............................67
Swimmer's Ear..............................68
Nosebleeds..............................69
Pinworms..............................69
Styes..............................70

Chapter 4: Digestive Disorders and Enemas..............................71
Diagnosing Digestive Disorders..............................71
Purpose of Enemas..............................72
Standard Enema..............................73
Retention Enema (Tea Enema)..............................75
Further Information on Preventing Dehydration..............................76
Recovery Diet..............................78
Antibiotics and Intestinal Disorders..............................80

Chatper 5: Fever..............................81
Diagnosing a Fever..............................81
Treatment..............................83
Fever and Enemas..............................85
Diagnosing the Severity of an Illness..............................85
Recovery..............................86

Chapter 6: Infectious Diseases..............................87
Diagnosis of Common Illnesses..............................88
Colds..............................89
Coughing..............................91
Wheezing..............................91
Flu..............................92
Pneumonia..............................93
Sinus Infection..............................94
Infected Ears..............................94
Strep Throat..............................96
Tonsils..............................98
Scarlet Fever..............................99
German Measles..............................100

Chicken Pox..100
Urinary Tract Infections..103
Whooping Cough..103
Cystic Fibrosis..104
How to Stop Passing the "Bugs" Around..105

Chapter 7: Antibiotics..107
Effective Use of Antibiotics...108
Penicillin...108
Ampicillin and Amoxicillin...109
Erythromycin...109
Allergy to Antibiotics..110
Administering the Antibiotics...110

Chapter 8: Allergies...113
Identification...113
Treatment...113
Allergies and Infants..115
Desensitizing Shots..116
Antihistamines and Decongestants...117
Emergency..117

Chapter 9: Dr. Denmark's Medicine Cabinet.....................119
Nonprescriptive Items...119
Prescriptive Items..125
Available Kitchen Items...127
Substitution Lists...128

Chapter 10: A Mother's Presence...135
Responsibility..139
Education..140
Economics...141
Johnny's Day..142
The Best?..145
Attitude..146
Relationships..147
Grandparents...148
Home...149
Expert Advice and Parenting..149

Chapter 11: Nutrition and Health Habits............................153
Nourishment..154
Protein...154
Starches..156
Vegetables...156

Fruit...156

Sweets...157

Drinks...158

Dairy Products...160

Calcium...161

Fats..161

Mealtime..162

Sample Menus...164

One-dish Meals...165

Complete Meal Bean Dishes.....................................169

Other Legume Recipes..170

Debra Ridings's Whole Wheat Bread.....................172

Routine..174

Sleep..175

Sunshine and Exercise...177

Guarding Our Children's Health....................................178

Chapter 12: What is Needful?.....................................181

Obedience...184

A Good Teacher...186

Papa..189

Back to the Basics...191

Time..192

Adolescents and Time...194

Jacob Abbott's Wisdom..196

Friendships...198

Clothing...203

Gender Distinctions...205

Boundaries..207

TLC..211

Dreams...214

Work...216

Teamwork..217

Ministry...219

Adversity...221

Christ..224

Recommended Parenting Resources..........................228

Chatper 13: Vaccinations...229

Chapter 14: Story Time..241

Generations..241

With Love...245
Reprieve...246
Answers...248
When All Else Fails...250
From Afar...253
Thank God!...255
Titus 2...259
Two by Two..265
Mother of Twelve...271
Coming Home..273

Epilogue...275

Biographical Sketch...279
Special Services and Studies...............................284
Memberships and Honors....................................284

Appendix I: Immunizations Source Charts.........287
U.S. Produced Vaccines from Aborted Cell Lines.........287
U.S. Produced Alternative Vaccines......................288

Appendix II: Shall We Watch a Movie?...............289

Appendix III: Bowmom's Maxims........................299

Index..303

Foreword
By Robert A. Rohm, Ph.D.

Little Rachael Anne Rohm, our first child, was born July 31, 1973. Neither her mother, nor I, knew what we were about to face. Children are a blessing from the Lord, but that does not make the task of parenting any easier. It is indeed a first-class challenge…especially when your firstborn arrives and you feel totally unprepared. The only real help comes from reading "baby books", listening to relatives and calling other trusted friends. In addition to all that, proper child rearing is a delicate issue with many people, especially new parents.

Rachael dominated our every waking and non-waking moment. When she cried, we jumped! We had heard that when a child cried, it had a need. It did not take her long to have a lot of needs! She seemed to never sleep, wanted to feed on demand, and was just irritable in general. We loved her dearly, but really questioned our ability in being up to the task of parenting her.

Then one day a lady family friend told us about this special, unusual pediatrician by the name of Dr. Leila Denmark. (Looking back, I can see that our friend understood our dilemma better than we did. We only understood the problem, but she actually understood the solution!)

We went to see Dr. Denmark. After an introduction and a few preliminaries, Dr. Denmark looked at us and said, "Did you move in with the baby, or did the baby move in with you?" She then proceeded to explain the importance of a schedule and routine and the fact that at times babies needed to cry in order to get exercise (provided they had been fed and were clean). I liked the way she spoke with certainty. Her wisdom, "horse sense," professional manner, caring attitude and compassion for child and parent alike sold us immediately. Needless to say, in time some marvelous changes began to occur.

As the years passed, we had three more children. Their first years were so different, so pleasant! It was the difference between day and night. We had learned so very much from this wise medical doctor. Bringing home and caring for newborns actually became a pleasant experience. In addition to all this, I know for a fact all of our children were a lot healthier, too. Rachael, who had often been sick with routine illnesses, began to be healthy. The other children were healthier as well. It is amazing how much money we were able to save in unnecessary health care costs.

Dr. Denmark has not only been a real friend to "little people" as she refers to them, but she has also been a lifeline to parents. Quite frankly, I do not know what we would have done without her.

As you read the wisdom contained in these pages, you will silently thank God for the excellent work Madia Bowman has accomplished. Her eight years in researching, writing, and focusing on Dr. Denmark's thoughts and philosophies will save you time, effort, and a lot of unnecessary heartache. Dr. Denmark is a very special person. Since she has recently passed the century mark in age, now seems to be a fitting time to put her excellent opinions and remedies in writing.

Read, enjoy, marvel, but most of all, apply. You and your child will be the winners for it. God bless you!

Dr. Robert A. Rohm
President, Personality Insights
Atlanta, Georgia

Acknowledgments

When I started this book our son David was a newborn. We celebrated his eighth birthday a week after the first edition was complete. God has good reasons for keeping the future a secret. If I had known the extent of this project or that David would have six younger siblings, I would never have attempted it.

Miraculously, the book was finished, and now a new edition is available. So many people have encouraged and helped. Marlene Goodrum shared this vision in its seed form, patiently deciphered my scribbling, and typed the earliest draft. Cathy Hoffer helped in a myriad of ways: proofreading, brainstorming, advising, and contacting publishers. Lynn Holman spent countless hours typing and revamping. I want to thank Mary Hutcherson (Dr. Denmark's daughter), Jennifer Simon, Julia Lee Dulfer and Janice White for reviewing, editing, and help with layout. My husband Steve also shared the vision and wrote Dr. Denmark's biographical sketch.

The work couldn't have continued had it not been for our older daughters, Malinda and Jessica, who looked after the little ones while I was writing. Jessica also helped put together the index. Katie Fearon and Sarah Pitts babysat when my daughters were unavailable. I cannot forget the moms who took the time to write the testimonials, many of which are included in chapter fourteen.

There were so many others who helped, advised, and encouraged: my brother Andy Linton, my mom Betty Linton, Traci Clanton, Nora Pitts, Tim and Windy Echols with Family Resource Network, Suzanne and Larry Miller, Creston Mapes, Jim Vitti, Paula Lewis, Gina Booth, Terri Lynn Fike, James

Demar, Luis Lovelace, and Helen Lin. My heartfelt thanks to Jerry White for being a wonderful friend and source of counsel (Proverbs 27:9). Without Gary DeMar of American Vision, this book might never have come to completion. He helped tremendously in the final stages of preparing the first edition for publication.

I very much appreciate the patience and support of our younger children as subsequent editions came along. While mother spent time editing, Steven, Esther, David, Joseph, Leila, Christina, Susanna, John and Emily all carried extra household duties. Esther, Leila and Christina bore the greatest responsibility in supervising meals and schoolwork. Thank you Leila, for functioning as my "right arm" and your willingness to type revisions. Steven, the new book cover for our English edition looks great!

Dad Bowman graciously relinquished his apartment for a few days so I could have a quiet haven to make final revisions. Jon Rogers also helped with interpreting Adobe, and the initial layout. Dr. Rhett Bergeron and my Uncle Jeff (Dr. Jefferson Flowers) consented to recommend substitutions for some of the hard-to-obtain medications. They were very generous with their time and expertise.

Joel and Judy Linton (our nephew and niece) have been an enormous inspiration. They are missionaries to Taiwan and have disseminated Dr. Denmark's methodology to a receptive Taiwanese public through Judy's own book. Judy's example and generous support from Jeanne and Greg Badgett paved the way for us to pursue a Mandarin translation of this publication.

Thank you, Jean Heidel, for translating *Dr. Denmark Said It!* into the beautiful Mandarin language. Eileen Li, our editor and dear friend, spent countless hours pouring over these pages, grappling with the nuances of English versus Mandarin vocabulary. To quote Judy's evaluation of the translation in progress, "Jean's personable, readable manner [coupled with]

Eileen's meaning corrections and stylistic perfections, your book will reach into the "A++ category."

Pastor Neil Brown has been an enormous help in furthering the Spanish translation of our manuscript. He and First Baptist Church of Woodstock, Georgia, provided financial support as well as introducing us to a unique mother/daughter translation team: Maria Calsada and Mayra Burns. We were blessed to have access to Mrs. Calsada's linguistic and cross-cultural understanding as well as her knowledge of medical terms. Mayra, we are grateful for your linguistic and formatting skills too. It has been wonderful and appropriate to have a young mother as part of the translating team. Thank you for persevering through significant health challenges, a relocation of your family and a difficult pregnancy. Congratulations on the newest baby, Burns!

Last, but not least, I cannot fail to thank God, my merciful heavenly Father, for the vision and resources to complete this book. He is the one who brought Dr. Denmark into my life and relocated her practice five minutes from our home. She cared for my children and helped me in countless ways for 32 years. I am grateful for her example, wisdom, and willingness to support this project. I will greatly miss her until we meet again.

None of us knows exactly what Heaven will be like; its joys are beyond all imagination. Yet on a very small scale, I believe there was a taste of Heaven under those spreading oak trees and tin roof on Mullinax Road. There, within a renovated farm house clinic, life was promoted and love displayed. Midst the chatter of mothers and children within its walls, a kind, patient voice was often heard asking: "Now who's the next little angel?"

Introduction

I would never claim that my methods are the only correct ones, nor presume to tell another physician that his advice was all wrong. In the final analysis parents must decide for themselves what they think is best for their child. However, I will say this—I have practiced pediatrics successfully for over seventy-five years. During that time I have found that these methods have worked for me and my patients. Suppose you asked me for directions for downtown Atlanta. I would tell you the roads I have taken to arrive there safely. In the same way I share with you my experience in caring for children.

—Leila Denmark

For over 75 years thousands of children were lovingly treated by Dr. Leila Denmark. Their concerned, confused and tired mothers benefited from her advice. They came away encouraged, admonished, with practical suggestions for tending ailing youngsters and wise counsel for living.

In our fast-changing culture, moms can become thoroughly confused by conflicting information. Modern child psychology, trendy pediatrics, and shifting views on nutrition contribute to frustrated parenting.

Dr. Denmark offered a breath of sanity in the midst of confusion. She encouraged mothers to "look for the obvious" and "use their own minds," thus guiding them through the maze of advice from so-called experts. Her counsel is not simply a reflection of the latest medical journal. Instead, her recommendations are largely based on decades of successful medical practice. Dr. Denmark's counsel is time tested.

I found that the hours I spent in Dr. Denmark's clinic were not only useful from the standpoint of receiving practical medical advice, but they afforded a fascinating glimpse into the past. Having grown up in the early part of the twentieth century, her perspective on family life reflects an earlier, perhaps healthier social era in America when more families looked to the holy Scriptures as their guide for life and practice.

In 1990 I determined to compile some of Dr. Denmark's medical wisdom. My original goal was to add an appendix to her book, *Every Child Should Have a Chance*. When approached about the project, she had another idea.

"Mrs. Bowman, you take what I've said and write it down. Add some of your own insights. You're the mother of five (now eleven) children. You know something. Write your own book." She paused thoughtfully, "Maybe you can help somebody." So that's what I've done.

Unless otherwise specified, all the medical advice contained herein comes directly from Dr. Denmark. Medications, treatments, daily routines, and diets are her recommendations. I've included a number of personal letters that attest to their practicality. In this edition, we have added two substitution lists for medications which are now difficult to obtain.

As for the child-rearing philosophy, it's my own, developed through the study of the Bible, books, excellent counsel, personal experience and numerous conversations with Dr. Denmark. I hope you will enjoy her words of wisdom appearing throughout the text. Quotes which are not footnoted come from recorded discussions with her.

I also hope that those who read these pages will be encouraged to look to the greatest physician, Christ Jesus, as He is revealed in the Bible. He is the one who blessed me with Dr. Denmark as mentor, and He is ultimately the only one who can bring true healing to body and soul. My prayer is that this book will indeed "help somebody."

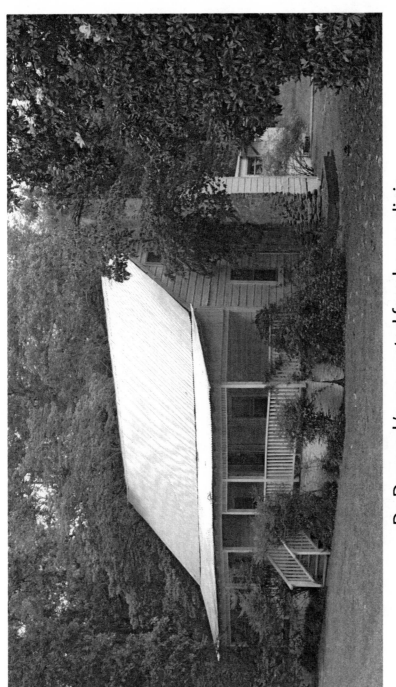

Dr. Denmark's renovated farmhouse clinic on Mullinax Road in Alpharetta, Georgia

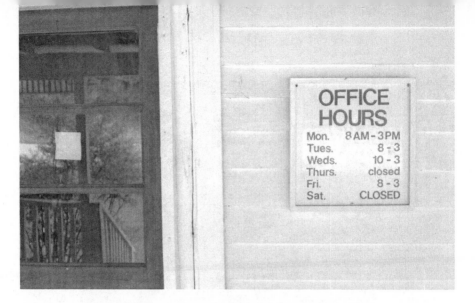

Office hours posted at the front door

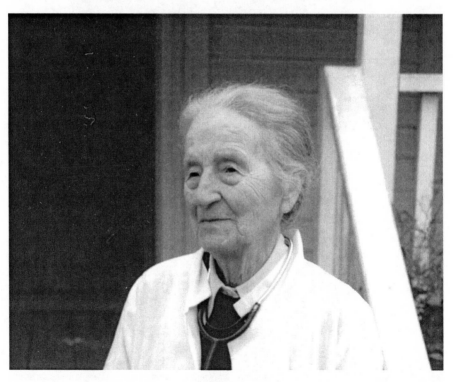

Dr. Denmark on her front porch

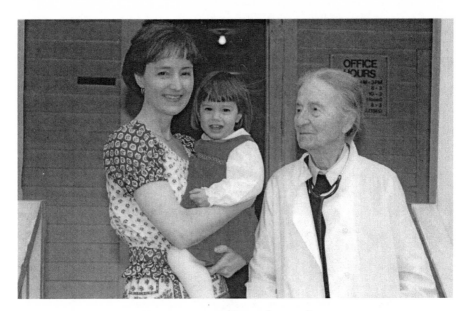

Dr. Denmark with author
and daughter Christina

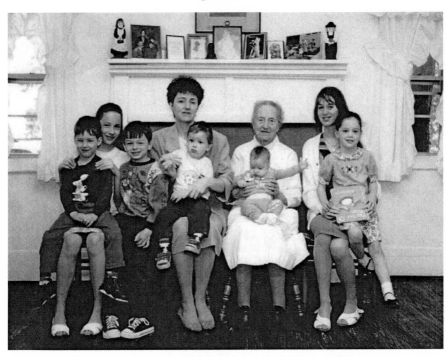

Young Bowman family with Dr. Denmark
in the patient waiting room

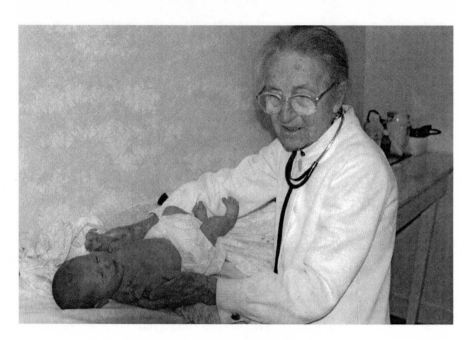

Examining a newborn

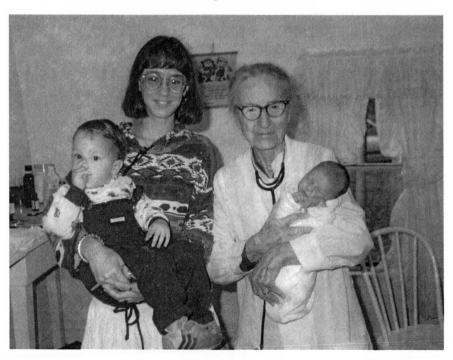

Posing with siblings: Malinda,
Joseph, and Leila

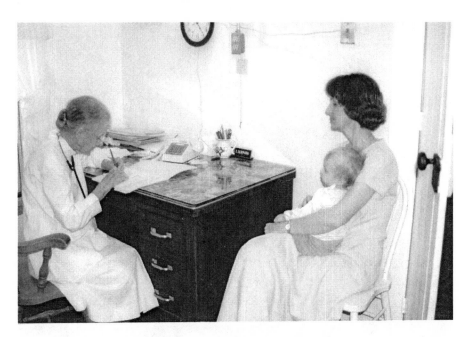

Filling out patient records

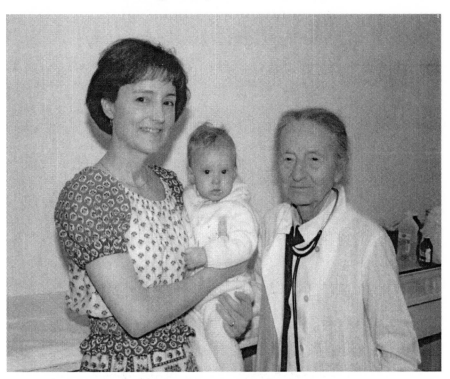

Author with baby Susanna

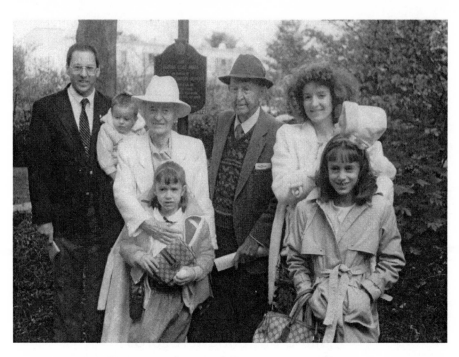

Denmarks and Bowmans after
the Shining Light Award ceremony

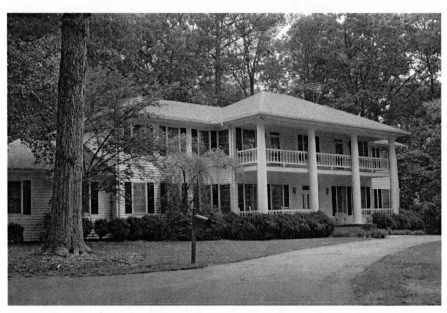

Denmark home on Mullinax Road
(next door to the clinic)

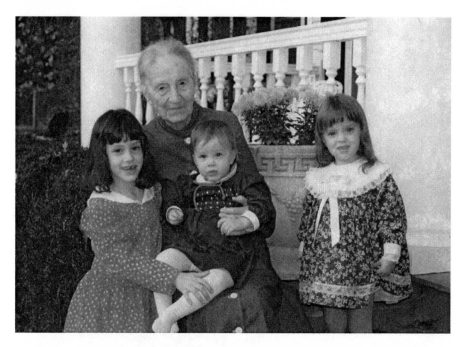

Sitting on the front steps with
Esther, Christina, and namesake Leila

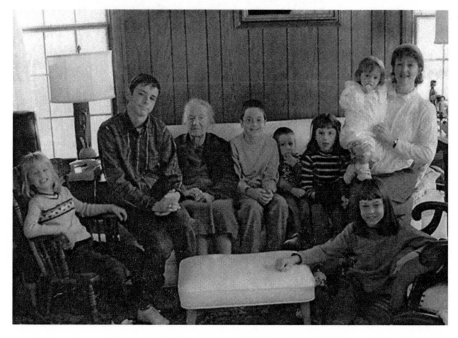

Gathered in the Denmark den

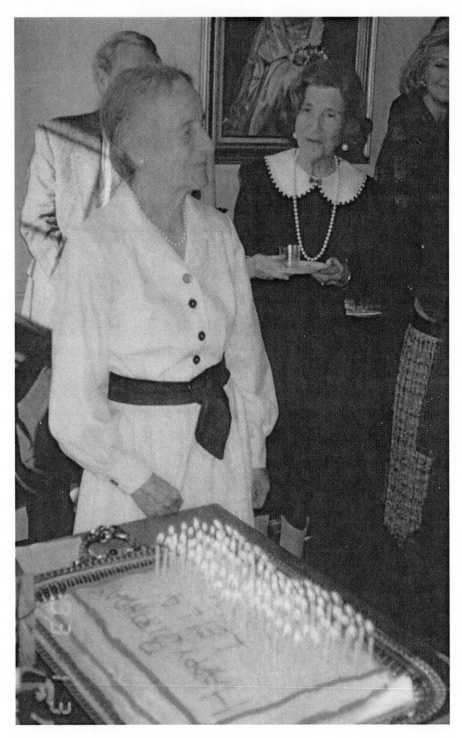

Happy 95th birthday

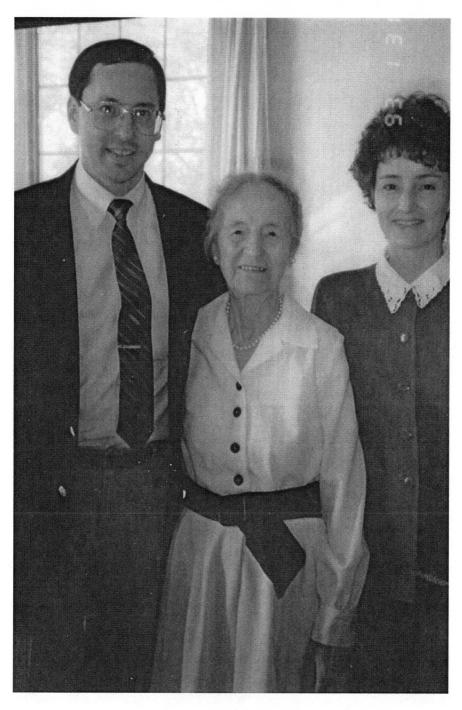

Posing with author
and husband, Steve

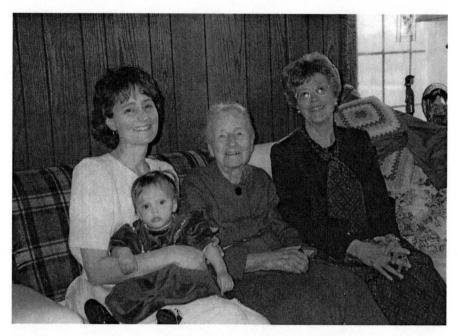

Visiting with fellow "Denmarker"
Gwendolyn Webb and baby Emily

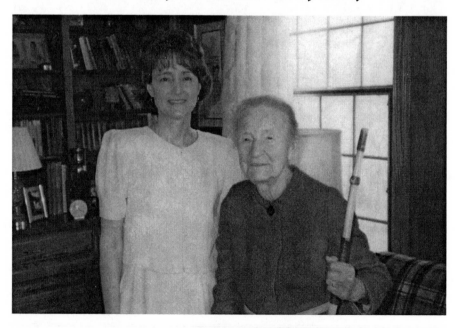

Author and Dr. D. holding her
well-known walking stick.

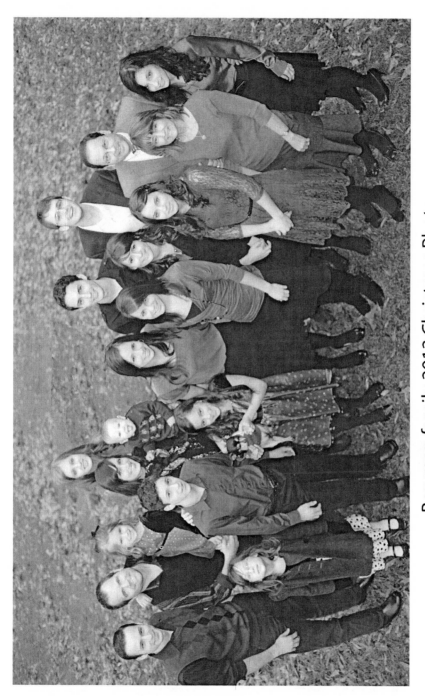

Bowman family 2012 Christmas Photo

❀ 1 ❧
Care of Infants

There is no more important job on earth than rearing children. The direction a person takes depends to a large extent on the training and leadership he has from birth through childhood, and even after becoming an adult. Our world desperately needs parents – parents who are willing to give their children the opportunity to grow and develop in keeping with their physical and mental capacity. We need parents who will take the time to help their children develop healthy bodies and souls, so as to enjoy full, happy and useful lives.

On January 9, 1980, a young woman sat in the waiting room of Dr. Leila Denmark's office holding her first child, a two-day-old baby girl.

The new mother's emotions ranged from bewilderment to awe to trepidation as she gazed at her daughter's tiny face. In her arms lay a great blessing ... and an overwhelming responsibility. Her own mother was thousands of miles away in a foreign country, unavailable for day-to-day counsel. She so wanted to be a good parent and do everything right.

Friends recommended Dr. Denmark. Could an 82-year-old pediatrician be that capable? Had she made the right decision in coming?

Dr. Denmark must have sensed her anxiety. "You see that little squirrel out in the tree? She has never been to a doctor or read a book, but she knows just what to do for her babies. She feeds them, keeps them clean and comfortable and away from people. It's not as complicated as people might make you think!"

Dr. Denmark spent over an hour with the young mother, patiently going over the basics of common-sense infant care. She left the office much reassured and empowered, never dreaming what an impact that appointment would have on her family. Years later, after having borne eleven children, she remembers and is thankful. I am that woman and I hope I can pass on to my readers the wise counsel I was blessed to receive.

A child is a precious gift, divinely given. Nothing is more helpless than a newborn, who is completely dependent on his parents' care. Actually, parenting begins before birth. At the moment of conception, a new child is created; and his health largely depends on the health of his parents and his mother's nutrition during pregnancy. A life of dissipation and addiction will inescapably and sometimes permanently affect the baby within. Mother is surely "eating and drinking for two" so she must beware what she puts in her body. Addictions to nicotine, alcohol, snuff, narcotics, and even caffeine will interfere with baby's health. Consuming too many dairy products can cause anemia in mother and affect her child. Mother should put away that which is harmful and consume only what is healthful out of love for her baby.

If a woman who has been involved in substance abuse finds out she is pregnant, the answer is not abortion, for her baby is already a living person, created in God's image. Instead, she should resolve to abstain from harmful substances and get help. Love for her pre-born child can often bring great change in a woman's life.

Pregnancy can potentially give birth to two new lives: baby's and mom's!

A healthy newborn is sleepy, happy, hungry, docile, cuddly, but —wow—what lungs! The advent of an infant into the home can bring a frenzied, sleepless, and trying time or be a precious experience filled with peace and wonder. A few principles of child care can make all the difference. New parents need wise counsel so that mother, father, and baby get off to the best start possible.

When I was a young doctor, I used to meet with new parents at the hospital after the baby arrived. Often grandparents came, too. The first thing I said to the mother was, "This baby has come to live with you, not you with the baby. He needs to be trained into a system. If you were building an important business, you'd have a system, and building a human being is the most critical thing on earth. You're going to die one day and leave this little creature here. If you haven't built him a way of life, somebody's going to kick him around. That's the reason our jails are so full today. Those people didn't have a chance because they didn't have parents who taught them a way of life.

The day that baby was conceived, everything was in one cell: its height, color, disposition, its whole life. If you took care of yourself during pregnancy—didn't drink, smoke, do drugs, or drink too much milk—at birth that baby is all it was meant to be. Now, if you don't feed him right and look after him properly until he's eighteen years old, he can never reach his full potential. This little baby has to have a system. There should be a time for everything.

You will have everybody on earth telling you how to rear your child. I'm telling you, your mother-in-law's telling you, all your neighbors are going to tell you how to do it. Listen carefully to what everybody says and respectfully reply, "Yes, ma'am; yes, sir." Then go home and do just what you think is best.

Newborn

Schedules

Demand feeding or feeding every two hours round-the-clock is often recommended for newborns. Many assume that demand feeding simulates the more "natural" and wholesome habits of the animal kingdom and human mothers that lived long ago. Dr. Denmark claimed that this assumption is wrong. Having grown up on a farm, at the turn of the twentieth century, she observed first-hand that animals had a rhythm to their eating habits based on their particular digestive systems. Her own mother, a farmer's wife, would never have had the time to nurse on demand. Her mother did not live at the frenetic pace many modern women tend to fall into. She took time to relax and nurse her babies. However, without modern refrigeration and labor-saving devices, a farmer's wife was too busy to nurse every time baby squeaked. Feedings had to be spaced so necessary chores could be completed. All family members needed their rest at night, so baby was trained to the rhythm of a happy, active household.

Demand feeding is likely to produce exhausted and depressed mothers, colicky babies, and chaotic homes. A good routine of eating and sleeping is vital for the health of the child and for family harmony. Milk meals need to be spaced sufficiently to allow time for the infant's stomach to empty before adding more milk.

The stomach is a small sack, and the food has to remain in the stomach and be mixed with the hydrochloric acid and pepsin and be digested before it is expelled into the gut to be mixed with the bile and pancreatic juices. After this process of digestion, the food is absorbed to supply the needs of the body. If we continue to add milk to the stomach without giving the milk that is in the stomach time to be digested and expelled, the stomach has to expand more and more because the stomach does not expel milk into the gut until it has been digested in the stomach. With the constant adding of milk, there would never be a time when all the milk in the stomach would have gone through the process of digestion; but the old would be mixed with the new. The only thing that could happen would be for the stomach to expand to accommodate all that was put in, or the undigested milk would have to be passed into the gut, or the baby would have to spit up to get relief. So we see that feeding a child every time he cries would create a serious problem.[1]

Upon returning from the hospital, a mother should put her newborn on a consistent schedule of eating and sleeping. This routine does not simply benefit parents or promote parental convenience. Scheduling is best for baby! Training a child to eat and live on a sensible routine is not only fundamental for his good health. It enhances the child's ability to live a productive life and promotes character development. The infant learns during his earliest days that he cannot expect to have every perceived need gratified instantly. The consistent routine builds a sense of security. He learns that he can depend on and trust his parents to meet his true needs at the appropriate time. The following schedule is recommended:

6:00 a.m.   Feed breast milk or formula; allow baby to sleep in an open room. Raise the window shades and leave the door ajar if there is no danger of a toddler harming the baby.

9:30 a.m.   Bathe (as needed).

10:00 a.m. Feed and put down for nap with door and shades closed. Assure quiet.

2:00 p.m.   Feed, leaving the room open.

6:00 p.m.   Feed and play with baby.

10:00 p.m. Feed. Change diaper; check to see if baby is all right. **Do not pick the child up or feed him until 6:00 a.m.**

Crying Infant

If a baby cries all the time and for no apparent reason, we know something is wrong and the cause should be explored. However, for an infant to be healthy and develop properly, it is critical that he spend a certain amount of time crying loudly. Crying is a natural way of expanding and strengthening his lungs and giving baby his necessary exercise. A newborn generally sleeps twenty hours out of 24. A healthy baby may spend up to four hours crying every day. That fussing can take place at one particular time of day such as evening hours, or baby may cry some before each feeding. With patience and persistence, he can be trained to fuss during daylight hours so everyone gets needed rest at night.

Before a child is acclimated to the above schedule, he will probably want to be fed during the night. A baby doesn't need to feed in the middle of the night. He should be getting all of his nutritional needs met during day feedings. If parents are consistent with the above schedule, most children become accustomed to it after a few days and will begin sleeping through the night.

Our children were usually trained to sleep through the night within ten days. Our first baby, Malinda, took four nights. Some infants take longer than others to train. If your baby is one of those ask yourself, "Am I following the schedule consistently? (Consistency is vital.) Is my baby positioned so that he feels secure (see pages 16-19)? Am I keeping his bedroom quiet? Do I need to exercise self-control and persevere a few more nights?"

Many mothers, including our oldest daughter, Malinda (who now has children of her own) find it easier to train their newborns to sleep through the night if baby is sleeping in a separate room from mom and dad. Try putting the crib in a safe, separate room, ensuring that toddlers do not have easy access to baby. Once, we discovered our adventuresome three-year-old had climbed into bed with his infant sister— not a safe scenario! Installing locks on the outside of nursery doors is not a bad idea.

Many experienced "Denmark moms" also recommend **keeping baby awake as much as possible between the six and ten o'clock feedings** so he is more likely to sleep through the night. Bring him into the living room and play gently with him. If it is not too noisy, this would be a good time for other family members to interact with him as well. Bear in mind, however, that a newborn will snooze off and on throughout the day.

Use your discretion, remembering that normal, healthy infants do cry even if nothing is wrong. Many things can wake a baby up. Check for fever, a stuffy nose, diaper rash, or abnormal bowel movements. Is the temperature of his room comfortable? Is baby gaining normally?

After ruling out the above, you might try giving him a little formula at ten o'clock after you nurse him. You may be tired and not producing enough milk in the evening. Mix one tablespoon of powdered formula with two ounces of sterile water (yielding two ounces of formula).

If he drinks the entire amount, feed him two and one-half ounces the next night after nursing. Continue increasing the amount every night by one-half ounce until he leaves a little in the bottle. An infant will not drink too much. Minor supplementing at his ten o'clock feeding may be all it takes to help baby sleep until six (see pages 10-12).

Babies need a lot of affection and I loved cuddling my babies, but as a new mother it was a tremendous relief to me to realize I didn't have to pick baby up every time she cried. I noticed that she fell asleep sooner at bedtime when I let her fuss a while (See pages 246-248, 251, 271-272).

Crying is a very important part of a baby's development. Babies must cry, and cry hard, to open up their lungs to full capacity. A pre-mature infant, baby with Down's syndrome, baby that is injured at birth, or a very weak baby may have trouble expanding his lungs to the normal capacity.

The child must learn at an early age that crying cannot get for him things that are not good for his physical or mental development. Babies cannot sleep all the time, and we must love them enough to hear them cry if it is necessary for their normal development and training. I say to mothers, "If you don't let this baby cry today, he may make you cry tomorrow."[2]

Feeding

Breast Feeding

Nurse your baby if possible. It contributes to the mother's and especially the baby's good health. A nursing mother should eat plenty of protein, whole grains and leafy, green vegetables and drink lots of water and soups (no milk or juice) and be happy.

Nurse your baby ten minutes on each side, burping him at the change-over and after nursing. When on the first breast, press the nipple of the opposite breast to keep its milk from flowing. Encourage sleepy baby to stay wakeful during nursing so he will receive maximum benefit. If he is very groggy, try flicking his little feet or talking to him. Undress him if he is too warm.

After nursing, wash the baby's saliva off your breasts with clear water (no soap), dry them, and put clean cotton fabric between the nipples and bra. The cleansing is especially important while your nipples are becoming acclimated to nursing. Washing helps prevent (or treat) cracked, sore nipples. Note that thrush in the infant's mouth can also produce soreness (see pages 21-22). If the nipples have become so badly cracked that there is actually a cut, you may apply Silvadene cream (see page 126) after each feeding. Rinse it off with clear water before the next nursing. The residual Silvadene will not hurt baby.

As baby grows and becomes more wakeful, he will empty the breast more quickly. After a few weeks, you will not need to time him ten minutes on each breast.

A contented mother nursing her baby is one of the closest things to heaven on earth, and I speak from personal experience. There can never be created an equal to this normal method, even if it is worked out on the most scientific basis. The security, the antibodies, the mother-child relationship, the human protein cannot be created in a laboratory.[3]

Some people think that frequent and prolonged nursing increases milk supply. No, that doesn't do it at all. I had a woman in here the other day who was nursing her baby every two hours around the clock. She was worn out and looked like heck. The baby looked like the wrath of God, and the husband was ready to leave home! She didn't need to nurse her baby every two hours. The way to make milk is to be happy, have a system, and love to do it.

Premature Infant

Many have asked if Dr. Denmark recommended putting a premature baby on the same four-hour feeding schedule. The answer is, "yes!" A preemie's stomach still takes the same amount of time to digest milk. Some mothers of premature infants who have used Dr. Denmark's feeding schedule do give their preemies one middle-of-the-night feeding until they reach their "normal" due date, at which point they drop the night feeding. (See pages 265-271)

If the baby is small and weak, one might think he should be allowed to nurse for a long time, but that is not true. The smaller and weaker babies are the ones that should not be worn out with long feeding periods. The longer they suck, the more air they swallow and the more colic they have.[4]

Note: We have found that the four-hour feeding schedule works beautifully for most children. Breast milk takes approximately three hours to digest.[5] When a mother nurses her baby ten minutes on each breast, burping and possibly changing diapers between, she will use 30-40 minutes. Add time for milk to fully digest, a little extra for baby to develop an appetite, and four hours have transpired.

If, however, you have consistently nursed on the four-hour schedule for some time, and your baby always seems desperately hungry a half-hour before the next feeding, try adding one extra feeding during the day. Try nursing at 6am–9am–1pm–4pm–7pm-10pm. This schedule preserves the morning nap time and night sleep hours while spacing other feedings closer together. After a few weeks you can transition back into the four-hour routine.

If your baby is still not happy even with an extra feeding, and **especially if he is not gaining well**, supplements are probably in order. Formula does take longer to digest, so it should always be given at four-hour intervals.[6]

Supplements

The amount of milk a baby consumes is determined by his individual needs. If a child is gaining well and seems content, don't be concerned about the sufficiency of your breast milk. If the baby isn't gaining well and you're worried about his not getting enough, you can weigh him before and after nursing. During the first two weeks, most babies should weigh three to four ounces more after nursing. When he is six weeks old, he should weigh approximately eight ounces more after nursing. Most children continue to drink approximately eight ounces until they are weaned if pureed foods are introduced at the proper time.

If your child isn't receiving enough breast milk, you should supplement with formula, but always nurse first. (Otherwise your breast milk will quickly dry up.) After nursing, offer him however many ounces of formula he is lacking. For example, if your three-week-old gains only two ounces after nursing, offer him approximately two ounces of formula at the first feeding. If he drinks the entire amount, increase it by one-half ounce at the next feeding. A baby won't drink too much formula. You can continue increasing the amount by half-ounces **until he leaves a little in the bottle**. That way you can be certain he's receiving all he needs.

Try a cow's milk formula first. If the baby spits up constantly, has eczema, diarrhea, or multiple ear infections, switch to a soybean formula (see page 12-13). Keep trying until you find one that works. Some formulas are too concentrated for a newborn. If you're using formula that is intended to be diluted with water, add a little more water than the directions indicate on the can until your baby is three months old. Instead of one can of water to one can of formula, use **one-and-one-half** cans of water to one can of formula. After your baby is three months, follow the directions on the can.

It is critical that the formula is warm and flows freely from the baby's bottle. If a baby exhausts himself sucking from the bottle, he may quit before he is full. You don't want him to have to suck longer than 15 to 20 minutes. Sucking too long on the bottle can also injure the epithelium of the tongue and mouth, rendering the mouth more susceptible to thrush. If you have any concern over the milk flowing freely enough from the nipple, you can make a cross cut at the tip with a razor blade. Each cut should be approximately one-sixteenth of an inch long. Hold the bottle firmly while baby is drinking and provide some resistance to his sucking motion so he can pull on the nipple as he would pull on a breast nipple.

Although my figure is on the petite side, breast feeding was never much of a problem with our first seven children. Contrary to what many think, the size of a woman's breasts has very little to do with her ability to breast feed.

When Christina was born (number eight), however, I was unable to produce all she needed and had to supplement. She never nursed aggressively, and finally at five months rejected the breast altogether. Initially, my reaction was disappointment and grief. Somehow I felt like a failure, but my attitude changed. Hey, I wasn't a failure. Breast feeding is ideal, and I had been willing but just not able. Anyway, Christina was such a healthy, jolly little creature. Thank God for supplements when we need them! Thank God for healthy babies!

A baby at the breast or bottle learns the importance of mother and this should be the happiest time of the day for mother and baby; it should always be quiet—never in a rush.[7]

Spitting Up

Every baby will spit up sometimes. However, excessive spitting up can be caused by too frequent feedings (See pages 4-5), a food allergy, or a weak esophageal gastric valve. If a child spits up water in addition to formula, it's a good indication that he has a weak esophageal gastric valve, a normal condition in an infant. He may do it frequently for eight months but will gain normally.

Spitting up only formula or breast milk may indicate a food allergy. Try changing the formula. As a nursing mother, you need to eliminate various foods from your diet to determine the cause. Play "detective" and watch baby for improvement as you eliminate particular foods. You may need to eliminate a food for up to two weeks to determine whether it is a problem. Common offenders are milk products, citrus, and chocolate.

Projectile vomiting, especially in males, is cause for serious concern. It's like an explosion—the entire meal returns, and you can detect a rise and fall in his stomach as he ejects the food. Consult a physician immediately.

It's nice when babies spit up. They don't have as many colds because nobody wants to hold them!

Colic

When a baby is fretful and unhappy for no apparent reason, crying constantly, often spitting up and showing signs of abdominal pain we say he is "colicky." Every normal infant needs to cry for limited periods of time, but this behavior is distinguished from the miserable, colicky baby.

Many colicky babies are born of mothers who smoked, drank or took drugs during pregnancy (these may include prescription drugs). It will take weeks for such infants to behave normally, as they were born "addicted" and need time to get over withdrawal symptoms. If mother discontinues the stimulants or drugs and nurses her baby, the shock will be lessened to the baby's system. On the other hand, if he is put directly on formula, within 24 hours, it is likely he will become stiff and irritable.

...this little baby is a dope fiend, nicotine addict, coffee addict, alcoholic, or whatever the mother is addicted to; and to be deprived of the drug he has had for nine months makes him a wreck. He is jumpy, cyanotic, and stiff; he vomits, spits up, is constipated or has frequent stools, cries, and cannot be consoled until he has time to get over nine months of dissipation...sometimes a mother has to take a drug to protect her against convulsions, hypertension, and many other conditions that have to be treated to save the mother, but we must remember that the baby is getting everything the mother gets, and it takes time for the baby to get off the drug.[8]

Colic can also be caused by the wrong formula, or baby may be allergic to something his nursing mother is eating. Try switching the formula or diluting it (See page 11 for instructions). If you are breastfeeding, try eliminating allergy producing foods from your diet for at least two weeks (milk products, citrus and chocolate are common offenders). Babies positioned on their backs are far more likely to be colicky (See pages 16-19). These infants gasp and swallow too much air.

Probably the most common cause of colic in infants is too frequent feedings. Milk meals need to be spaced four hours apart to give the stomach time to digest food and pass it to the intestines before more food is added. Too frequent feedings cause indigestion, stomach pain and often spitting up.

If an infant is in pain, he will often make sucking motions. These are instinctive for an infant in any kind of distress. Mothers interpret the sucking motions as genuine hunger, so baby is fed again. Baby will drink more because he thinks sucking will stop the pain. Instead of resolving the pain, the new feeding increases it and we now have a colicky baby who keeps crying and sucking and crying.

In most cases, positioning a colicky baby on his tummy and putting him on a good schedule where meals are spaced sufficiently will eliminate the problem (See pages 4-5 and Index Colic).

I have found that demand feedings are very bad…the more often the baby is fed, the more he cries because his stomach is not empty when new food is added, making proper digestion impossible, and resulting in a very distended and painful stomach.[9]

Weight Gains

All newborns lose about eight ounces the first few days but should regain their birth weight after one week. From then on, infants usually gain one ounce daily until they are 12 weeks old (approximately five pounds). After that they drop down to gaining a half-ounce daily. At five months most infants have added approximately seven pounds to their birth weight.

Some healthy children will gain more and others not quite so much. The main things to watch for are a gradual gain and a happy baby. If there is no gradual weight gain, something is wrong and this problem should be solved as soon as possible. Supplements may be in order. (See pages 10-12)

Don't be too surprised or anxious if your baby doesn't look just like your neighbor's child. Your infant may have inherited your body type or that of your husband. After all, "You get apples off apple trees."

One of the finest babies I ever had wouldn't drink over three ounces at a time. Babies do have individual needs. Consistent weight gain is what a mother should look for.

Postpartum

For your own sake as well as your infant's, don't be in a hurry to get back to a full schedule after giving birth. If you can get some help with household duties, take advantage of it. Rest as much as you can for at least two weeks to give your body a chance to recover. If you're nursing, you need to let your milk get established. Staying quietly at home is best for both mother and baby.

When my child was born, I stayed in the hospital for two weeks. Then I went home, and somebody looked after me for two weeks. After that I took it kind of easy for a while. Maybe in the old days we overdid the recuperation period, but I do believe if you've been pregnant nine months you need some rest. You've lost some blood. Your abdominal muscles are weak, and everything is out of line. I think a mother should go slowly for about a month after delivery, especially if she plans to nurse.

Too much company and too much talk have been the downfall of many a helpless baby. These two—mama and baby—should be permitted to live together quietly and have a chance to get acquainted before either has time to get upset.[10]

If a mother gets up the day the baby's born and plans a banquet, she's weak, worn out, and likely out of sorts. If she wants to nurse, she must be happy. I think postpartum should be a time of peace. A woman needs time to get established before she tries to take over the whole shop again.

Positioning the Infant

Infants should always be placed on their stomachs for the first five months. They are safer and feel more secure in that position. An infant placed on his back flails his arms because he's afraid of falling. For months he has been enfolded in his mother's womb, but on his back, his limbs move too freely, so he feels insecure. He becomes startled, gasps, and takes in air that creates colic.

Leaving a baby on his back is potentially fatal. There is a constant danger that a child may spit up and asphyxiate himself if he's lying on his back. On his stomach, he's in no danger of choking on vomit. Towels placed under the sheet will absorb vomit, and the baby won't aspirate it into his lungs (see Furniture Use, page 19).

All of the baby's body systems work better on the stomach, and nothing drains properly on his back. It is easier for him to have bowel movements and pass gas. Back positioning contributes to sinus, respiratory and ear infections. Eustachian tubes cannot drain as well, so fluid builds up behind the eardrums and often leads to infection. Unfortunately many physicians will then insert tubes to drain the fluid (see pages 95-96).

An infant is better able to exercise his neck, shoulder and arm muscles while on his stomach. He will probably crawl sooner and longer. Crawling is critical to a child's mental as well as physical development.

Tummy sleeping also helps the child develop a nicely shaped head. Putting him on his side may cause a lopsided shape to his head. A child positioned on his back typically develops a broad face and a head that is flat on the back. If the infant is held a lot, the back of the head will look better but his face will remain more broad. Baby's face is nicely shaped by sleeping on his cheeks (See pages 252-253).

I've practiced medicine for over 75 years, and I've never had a crib death. I tell mothers, "The minute that baby's born, don't ever leave it on its back except to nurse it." [see Sudden Infant Death Syndrome, pages 232-234]

Years ago, mothers commonly placed infants with Down's syndrome on their backs. Babies with Down's have respiratory problems, and mothers were afraid they would smother on their faces. This was the wrong thing to do. The babies' heads would become flat and respiratory problems aggravated. Life expectancy with Down's syndrome was seldom over four years.

In my practice I never lost a baby with Down's syndrome. I always instructed the mothers to place the infants on their stomachs and have their tonsils and adenoids removed so they could breathe easier [See pages 98-99].

Clearly Dr. Denmark's advice on positioning infants flies in the face of the present "back-to-sleep" campaign pushed by so many hospitals and pediatricians. It grieves and frustrates me that young mothers are being persuaded by this propaganda. My children lived almost exclusively on their tummies (when they weren't being held) for the first twelve weeks. They slept, played, were bathed, diapered, dressed, and swaddled in that position. Dr. Denmark had long since demonstrated to me how to swaddle them and change their diapers while they were lying on their stomachs.

Swaddling makes baby feel snug and secure. The only time I refrained from swaddling my newborns, was when the weather was so hot that even the thin receiving blanket caused them to sweat.

Spread a receiving blanket on a smooth surface. Fold back one corner of the blanket and place baby **chest down** on it with his face on the folded portion. He should be in a crouching position, with his hands close to his cheeks, elbows bent. Next, fold back the opposite corner over his feet and tuck the other corners snugly around his body. Make sure his ability to breathe is not inhibited by the blanket. This method of swaddling enables baby to push up with his hands and exercise his neck and shoulder muscles when he is in bed.

If you are taking your infant outside on cold days, the folded corner of the blanket can be unfolded and flipped over baby's head to keep him warm. I would never cover baby's face with any-thing but a light receiving blanket and only when he is being carried.

Diapering a newborn on his stomach is really not a challenge. In some ways, it is easier to clean him in that position! When I did need to turn him over to clean his front or care for his umbilical cord, I would clasp his forearms and hands together against his chest to keep them from flailing and gently turn him over, keeping his hands together as I treated him.

When you are holding your newborn, don't let his arms flail around. Swaddle him and cuddle his tummy against your shoulder, chest, or forearm so he will feel safe.

The "back-to-sleep" campaign was in full swing by the time our youngest, Emily, was born. I remember watching her sleeping contentedly on her stomach and silently thanking God for the wise advice I had received.

Furniture Use

Infant swings and modern car seats unfortunately are not good for the spine. The cartilage between the vertebrae is particularly soft in a newborn's back, and he shouldn't be allowed to hunch over in the early months. It's best to keep him in his crib at home, spending minimal time in a car seat, especially before five or six months of age.

Making baby's bed properly is important. Spread four towels on the crib mattress and stretch a sheet tightly over them. This kind of surface contributes to proper breathing and absorbs fluid. **Never put your baby on a fluffy or furry-textured surface that might inhibit his breathing.** Nor should you place him on a carpet even with a blanket beneath him. Carpets contain a host of allergens, and babies can develop nasal congestion and ear infections from them.

Quietness

A newborn may not always appear to be sensitive to noise. In reality, he is very much affected by it. His eardrums are thin as tissue paper, and any sound he previously received through the amniotic fluid was muffled.

You'll want to protect your infant from unnecessarily loud noises, especially respecting sleep time. Keep the room as quiet as possible and allow a minimum of visitors, particularly during the first five months. Turn off the TV and the radio. If there's a telephone in the room, turn off the ringer.

It is unfortunate when mothers are in a hurry to take their infants into public. They need a quiet life away from the bustle of the outside world, particularly during those first five months. Exposing them to crowds increases the probability of their becoming sick, which can interfere with the rapid growth that is crucial at this time.

This new little life should be permitted to take the shocks gradually...The baby should be treated like the [American] Indians used to treat their babies, or like the cat treats her kittens—he should be hidden away for the first few weeks of life until he can get a good start.[11]

A little newborn has few immunities. If you take him to church and put him in the nursery on Sunday, I'll probably see him on Wednesday. Why? Because somebody brought a sick baby to the nursery and he was coughed on.

Sunshine

By the time your baby is two weeks old, take him outside for about five minutes a day. Lift his shirt and let the sun shine on his back. It will satisfy his requirement for vitamin D.

Jaundice

When the skin or the whites of the eyes seem unusually yellow in color, a child may be considered jaundiced. If your baby appears jaundiced, first check the color of his stools and urine. White stools and tea-colored urine mean no bile is coming through the bile duct. He needs the immediate attention of a physician. Normal urine and stools indicate your baby is probably just fine and needs no treatment. Sunlamps are not necessary, and he should not be taken off the breast. As indicated above, take him outside for a little sunshine on clear days.

A newborn can become jaundiced if the mother is anemic during pregnancy. The oxygen he received came through her blood via the placenta. If she was anemic, the oxygen level was low, and the child had to build as many red blood cells as possible in order to pick up whatever oxygen was afforded him. His system manufactured far more red blood cells than he needed after birth. The extra cells are then destroyed, causing jaundice, which usually disappears after a few days.

Anemia in pregnancy is commonly caused by overconsumption of dairy products (See pages 160-161, 156).

Pacifiers and Thrush

Babies should not be given pacifiers; it's much better for them to suck their fingers or thumbs. Those who use pacifiers may develop a fungus called thrush. White in color, it looks like curdled milk and covers the tongue, throat, cheeks, and roof of the mouth. In some cases it will spread to the buttocks and fingernails.

Breast nipples are soft and gentle. Sucking the rough rubber of a pacifier, interferes with the epithelial cells in the baby's mouth and can cause growth of the fungus that produces thrush. If just the top of the baby's tongue looks white and other parts of his mouth don't, he probably doesn't have it. He may simply be sleeping with his mouth open.

To treat thrush put nystatin suspension (see page 126) on a Q-tip and rub it on the insides of the cheeks, roof of the mouth, and under the lips after each feeding.

Never use water in a bottle as a pacifier. If your drowsy baby keeps sucking and you keep filling the bottle, excess water can dilute the baby's electrolytes (see page 158).

Dr. Denmark objected to the underlying mindset behind using pacifiers. She claimed that most parents who depend on pacifiers follow a pattern. They typically are not problem solvers. They stick a pacifier in baby's mouth to shut him up and will let him have other things that are not good for him simply because they don't want to hear complaints. Mothers should never pacify or give in to children's demands against their best interest. They should love them enough to refuse to comply when necessary and truly help children solve their problems.

A pacifier is a dirty thing. It is put down in places one would never put a toothbrush and then placed back in the baby's mouth. There are germs and fungus in the house, so many pacifier babies have thrush and diarrhea. A pacifier is nasty, but it does help the economy, and the doctor needs a job!

It seems to me that all "pacifier mothers" look alike, and they have the most insecure babies…[Some have suggested] that we take pacifiers away gradually. The answer to that comes from a story about one of my little patients who said he was going to cut off his puppy's tail. He told me he was going to cut off just a little piece each day so it would not hurt so bad.

I would say the way to deal with children is to do the things for them that are best now, and never bring the subject up again. The best way to stop this awful thing is to throw the pacifier in the trash and let the baby cry for awhile—then the show is over.[12]

Bathing

Bathe your baby with warm (not hot) water and soap that does not leave a residue. You can test the temperature of the water with your elbow. A newborn may be positioned tummy down on a table covered with a thick towel in a draft-free room and sponged off. Apply soap gently all over his body (head included.) Mother can lift the arms gently one at a time to wash, turning the head from side to side, and then lift his head up a little to clean his neck, all the while keeping him on his abdomen.

Rinse thoroughly with clear water. You can touch your tongue to his skin to taste for a soapy film. After his skin is soap free, dry him with gentle pats and refrain from using baby oils, powders or creams. These are unnecessary, can cause rashes, and make baby feel chilled. The chilling effects of a greased body can actually cause a lowering of white blood cells, rendering the infant more susceptible to infections.

Eyes and ears should not be cleaned with anything other than a bath cloth. If cotton swabs are used in the ear, wax or other substances could be forced back into the ear canal and cause trouble.

If there is a little mucus in the nose that is causing an obstruction, twist a small piece of cotton wet in sterile water into the nose, taking care not to insert it too far. Rubber syringes should never be used as they tend to cause mucus membranes to swell, producing congestion. Crying actually helps clean out baby's nose.

The vulva should be cleaned with sterile water using a small piece of cotton, never a cotton swab. Boys are easier to clean if they have been circumcised. Just wash the male genitals as other parts of the body are washed. If a baby boy has not been circumcised, then extra effort needs to be made to keep him clean to prevent infection.

It is better not to bother the umbilicus unless there is some discharge. It should be cleaned with a sterile piece of cotton, never covering the cord with adhesive dressing, but leaving it open to the air until it heals. Fold your baby's diaper so it does not cover his umbilicus while it is healing.

Clothing

After bathing your baby, dress him in soft, comfortable, absorbent clothing (preferably linen or cotton). Again, keep him on his stomach while you are diapering and dressing him. Make sure the diaper does not cover the umbilicus until it has healed.

Lift baby's head and slip the garment completely and quickly over his head so he can breathe freely. Then arms can be put through the sleeves. Ideally, all clothing worn by baby in the first three months should be fastened in the back if there are snaps or buttons. That way they do not rub against his stomach and make him uncomfortable. Sometimes, the garments work if they are put on backwards. The first gown that our Malinda wore to Dr. Denmark's office was a cotton gown with snaps down the front. Dr. Denmark showed me how to slip it on backwards for Malinda's greater comfort.

Unless the weather was very hot, I always used soft cotton T-shirts under cotton gowns in those first few months. If your baby sweats, he is overdressed and uncomfortable. Perspiring will release salts and oil from his skin and he will not feel clean. He obviously won't feel comfortable if the room is too cold either.

As young parents, we lived in a home with no air conditioning. During hot summer months, I dressed my infants simply in a cotton T-shirt and diaper. I didn't even use a receiving blanket, but was careful to place baby on his tummy. In later years, we moved to an air-conditioned house. At that time, my newborns ordinarily wore a T-shirt, gown, diaper, and socks. They were swaddled with a cotton receiving blanket depending on the weather. Use common sense and pay attention to the temperature of your baby's environment. Cover him with extra blankets if he needs them, and put a hat on his head if you take him outside on chilly days.

During the first six months of a baby's life a mother should choose clothes that are simply soft and comfortable. At six months, there is a definite change. At this stage, clothing must allow the child freedom to crawl.

At one year, gender distinctions become important. A little boy seems to know he's a boy and a girl knows, or seems to know, she's a girl. When she is dressed in a beautiful dress, she will show a marked feeling of pleasure. She likes to look in the mirror and admire herself. A little boy seems to throw his chest out when he is dressed like a boy and he has a boyish haircut.

At one year, if a male child is dressed like a girl and is made to wear long hair, typically he develops an attitude. He often becomes negative and destructive, wanting to prove to the world that he is certainly a tough boy regardless of his effeminate hair and clothes.

If we are around him very long, we will soon think he is demon-possessed... I have had the opportunity to follow these children from birth to adulthood and they never seem to get over the experience.[13]

Our little daughters loved bows and frills. Nothing caused more excitement than the Martha's Miniatures dresses their grandma purchased from the wholesale merchandise mart. These even had tiny bells sewn in the petticoats. On special occasions I often curled their hair around pink sponge rollers. Sunday mornings and especially on holidays, there was much dancing, swirling of skirts, jingling and bouncing ringlets.

It was easy to see that young girls have differing degrees of delicacy. Between Sabbaths, Leila paid little attention to her attire, happily romping outside and often coming back in with disheveled hair and grimy feet. Christina, on the other hand, was Miss Fastidious. She dressed carefully; constantly brushed her smooth, nut-brown locks; always wore shoes; and hesitated even to plant seeds in the garden. "I don't want to get my fingurs durty!"

Feet and Shoes

Every baby is born with crooked feet. They turn in or out depending on how he was positioned in his mother's womb. Typically, a child born with turned-in feet will walk sooner than one born with turned-out feet. Except in extreme cases such as clubbed feet, they will straighten out by themselves and need no orthopedic care. Baby really doesn't need shoes in the early months. He needs to use his feet, and it's easier for him to walk if he's barefooted.

Our Jessica's feet turned in considerably when she was a newborn. We were living overseas at the time and were advised by an orthopedist to put her feet in special shoes and braces. Later Dr. Denmark looked at her feet and reassured us that they were within the normal range. We followed Dr. D's advice and they straightened out with no problems. (At the writing of this edition, Jessica is training to run a marathon!) Our other children seldom wore shoes in their early years.

When I first started practicing medicine, we spent a world of money on night splints and special shoes. I found that if left alone, by age two most babies' feet would straighten out by themselves. If they're not straight by then, I have the mother buy roller skates and let baby skate a few minutes a day. It's a great way to train the feet to toe straight ahead.

My own grandchild didn't own a pair of shoes until he was one and a half. I went to see him one time, and he said to me, "Dr. Leila, I'm so proud of my little black shoes!"

Diaper Rash

Mild diaper rash appears as a slight redness. More severe rashes are fiery red and pimply and may even have blisters similar to those of a burn. Its three most common causes are antibiotics, alkaline urine (often a result of drinking juice), and allergic reaction. A severe rash is the result of an allergic reaction developing into a fungal infection.

When you change diapers, wipe baby's bottom with a wash cloth rinsed in warm water and wrung out. At bath time take care to rinse soap thoroughly from his diaper area.

Even a mild diaper rash is uncomfortable and can worsen, so it should be treated immediately. Try removing the diaper and allowing more air to get to the baby's skin. (You will have to change bedding frequently.) Also try to determine the cause of the allergic reaction that is producing the rash. Possible causes might be a particular detergent used to wash the diaper, or a food you're eating that the baby is reacting to through your breast milk. Don't give the baby any juices or too much fruit.

If you are using disposable diapers, you may need to switch to another brand. Consider using cloth diapers. Disposables are very air proof and keep the skin at a higher temperature than cloth diapers do, thereby contributing to fungus growth.

For a severe diaper rash, indicating a fungal infection, keep the area as dry as possible and apply nystatin topical powder(see page 126) three times a day. If the skin becomes raw and/or blistered, use Silvadene cream (see page 126) three times a day in addition to the nystatin. Apply the cream first and then sprinkle powder on top. (Common diaper rash ointments and creams can actually cause a severe rash to become worse.)

Teething

Many generations of American women have believed in "teething" as an intermittent condition needing attention and treatment. We are told that it can cause illness, fever, excessive pain and serious irritability. My great-grandmother, Lottie Witherspoon Bell, had baby Henry's gums lanced by a physician to reduce what she thought was pain from teething.

Dr. Denmark rejected this notion of teething. She said, "A child actually begins to teethe five months after conception and continues to do so for approximately eighteen years with no serious symptoms other than minor discomfort from erupting teeth." If your baby is truly sick, don't blame it on "teething." Look for another cause.

Recently our daughter Emily mentioned slight soreness in the back of her mouth. We also noticed a small flap of skin on her gum: twelve-years molars were coming through. It's clear that she is still teething!

Three Months
Schedules

6:00 a.m. Nurse.
9:30 a.m. Bathe (as needed).
10:00 a.m. Nurse and feed. Nap.
2:00 p.m. Nurse and feed. Play time.
6:00 p.m. Nurse and feed. Put to bed.
10:00 p.m. Nurse and put to bed for the night.

At 12 weeks you may notice your child stays awake longer, doesn't cry as long, and has begun drooling. Drooling is an indication that the child's saliva now contains ptyalin, the enzyme that enables him to change starch into sugar. It's time to begin slowly introducing pureed foods into his diet. The drooling stops when he learns to swallow his saliva. If his nose is stopped up, he may drool indefinitely.

The nursing schedule remains the same (6—10—2—6—10), but you may now offer **puréed** foods after nursing at 10—2—6. Try one new kind of food at a time, and observe the infant over the next 4–7 days for any signs of allergic reaction. During that time give him one-fourth teaspoon of the new food per meal, increasing each day until two tablespoons are given at 10-2-6.

If no reaction occurs you can assume there is no allergy. Now add another new food, one-fourth teaspoon at a time, increasing the amount to two tablespoons over a 4–7 day period. It's a safe way to introduce your baby to a large variety of foods, and you will detect any allergies early.

Should an allergic reaction occur, write down the particular food that caused it and a description of the reaction. It might manifest itself as a rash, diarrhea, asthma, eczema, vomiting, hay fever, a clear running nose, or excessive crying. Any abnormal condition should be recorded. Try the food in question one month later and check for a similar reaction. Introduce the food three times at one-month intervals. If the reaction occurs each time, you may assume that the child has a lifetime allergy to it.

Until they become acclimated to its new texture, many infants spit out most of the food. Some babies are easier to feed than others, but in any case be patient and keep trying. Have fun and enjoy the new experience with him.

Rice cereal mixed with breast milk or formula is good to start off with. Next introduce puréed bananas, apple sauce and a good protein (See page 33). After a protein, try a vegetable such as green beans or carrots.

Whenever you add a new food, mix it with the ones you have already tested. Babies are accustomed to the warm, sweet taste of breast milk or formula, so will more likely accept the purée if it is served warm and sweetened with fruit.

After a baby has been introduced to the above variety of food types (starch, bananas, cooked fruit, protein, vegetables), mom can vary the foods within each category. Instead of rice cereal, try oatmeal; instead of string beans, try spinach, etc. **Give baby as much of the "mush" as he wants.** You may be surprised at how much he will begin to eat.

Commercially produced baby food is fine (See page 33). If you make it at home, be sure it is well pureed and boiled for three minutes before serving.

Always offer the breast before food. **Bottle feedings come after food.** If you're supplementing your breast milk, nurse first, give pureed foods second, and bottle feed last. That order is more conducive to success. A supplementing mother should mix as much formula with the pureed food as possible.

Preemies usually catch up developmentally, but initially may be somewhat delayed. Often, it is wise to wait a few extra weeks before introducing pureed foods to a preemie. A baby born four weeks premature may need to wait an extra month and start puree at four months instead of three. Mothers should watch for signs of drooling, indicating that baby's digestive system has developed to a point where it is ready to process pureed foods (See page 270).

Baby food has done more for little people than anything except immunizations. Until about 75 years ago, mothers chewed for their children. The baby ate everything off her plate. Then we learned about germs, and mothers quit doing it. Babies couldn't chew for themselves and didn't get the nutrients they needed. So many developed scurvy, rickets, sprue— all kinds of deficiency diseases. People began to rub Campbell's vegetable soup through a sieve, and it worked like magic. One poor old man, a Mr. Clapp (I went hiking with him once in the Smokies), had a sick wife who couldn't digest food well, so he began sieving and canning it for her. He got the idea of making baby food that way and selling it. Then we went to "heaven"!

Homemade Baby Food

Dr. Denmark's baby-food plan worked wonderfully for all of our 11 children. Mixing the various food types with plenty of fruit as a sweetener is an excellent way to ensure that baby receives a balance of all the necessary nutrients. The mixture may sound disgusting, but our infants loved it and thrived on it.

When my babies were eating small amounts, I used commercial baby food for convenience. Dr. Denmark assured me that it was fine if it was the right kind (See page 33). However, anyone who has priced it at the grocery store knows the expense involved in using it regularly. After my babies were eating more, I normally made my own. The following tips may be helpful.

Invest in a good food processor or blender. There is no doubt our Cuisinart saved us thousands of dollars. Generally, food processors are better at pureeing meat. Blenders usually yield a smoother consistency. Our Emily was so particular about texture that I switched from a Cuisinart processor to a Cuisinart blender. It worked very well for all the foods I used.

Make sure all food is well-cooked and mixed with enough water to yield a smooth consistency when pureed. I usually made mine slightly thicker than the store-bought variety. Most babies don't like lumps and can choke on large ones. Be sure to blend or strain them out. Use well-ripened, sliced bananas.

Avoid using salty or spicy foods. I purchased salt-free items if I used canned foods and removed home-cooked vegetables before adding salt for the rest of the family. Make sure all food is fresh. Don't keep it in the refrigerator too long. **When in doubt throw it out.** Babies' stomachs are especially sensitive to bacteria. It's probably best to boil it just before serving, especially for young infants.

Some mothers make a week's worth of food at a time and freeze it in ice cube trays until needed. Others fix a couple of days' worth and keep it in the refrigerator. I generally made enough for three or four meals, pureeing the same food I had cooked for the rest of the family. Use whichever system you find most convenient.

Four Months

Schedules

If a child starts with pureed foods at 12 weeks according to Dr. Denmark's system, his consumption should increase rapidly. Now, he's ready to start a three-meal schedule. Space meals 5-1/2 hours apart for proper digestion (puree takes longer to digest than milk). Nurse before each feeding.

7:00 a.m.   Nurse and feed.*
9:00 a.m.   Bathe (as needed) and put down for a three-hour nap.
12:30 p.m. Nurse and feed;* play in the afternoon (no scheduled nap).
6:00 p.m.   Nurse, feed,* and put to bed (should sleep until morning).

*Any necessary bottle feedings should be given after pureed foods.

Breakfast
- 2 tablespoons fruit
- 3 tablespoons protein
- 3 tablespoons starch
- 1 banana

The tablespoon measurements indicated above are of **puréed** foods. All foods should be well blended, mixed together, boiled for three minutes and served warm. It is better to serve food to baby right out of the pot, reducing the risk of contamination.

Lunch
- 2 tablespoons fruit
- 3 tablespoons protein
- 3 tablespoons starch
- 3 tablespoons vegetables
- 1 banana

Supper
- Same as lunch

Acceptable proteins are lean meat, eggs, and black-eyed peas. Other beans may be used occasionally, but black-eyed peas are the superior legume because of their high protein content.

Leafy or green vegetables are best to use because of their high iron content. Other vegetables may be interspersed with them. Commercially produced baby food is fine, but always purchase unmixed varieties. Combination foods contain too much starch. For example, buy beef and carrots in separate jars, not as beef stew.

The amounts of food listed on the previous page are for the average appetite. Some children will eat more and some less per meal. **Make sure baby gets as much as he wants of the mix-**

ture with the same proportions that are listed. There should be a little food left in the bowl indicating he is full and has had enough. Your child shouldn't have juice or any other beverage.

When our John was an infant, he had a voracious appetite and consumed nearly double the amounts that are listed for each meal. We were going through a tight time financially and cut back on meat consumption. He was a vigorous, happy baby and ate "buckets" of black-eyed peas!

Naptime

At four months a baby no longer needs a scheduled afternoon nap. He may catnap on his own in the playpen or car seat but should begin weaning himself from sleeping in the afternoon. Encourage him to stay awake by keeping him in the living room or kitchen so he can watch family activity and play with his toys.

Weaning our babies off that afternoon nap usually took some time, but gradually they became acclimated to taking just one long nap in the morning.

Five Months
Food, Schedules, Sleep

Diet, mealtime, and sleeptime are identical to the four-month schedule, but now begin giving him small sips of water from a cup after each meal. There's never any need to give it in a bottle. It takes practice, but a baby can learn to drink from a cup at an early age. (He may cough and sputter a little at first.)

When my babies were learning to drink from a cup, I usually trained them with a clear glass or plastic one so I could see when the water met their lips. After they were drinking easily, we often switched to a "sippy cup" so they could drink on their own without much spilling.

Don't give a child mashed or whole food until enough molars have developed for proper chewing (usually between 24-28 months: development is individual). Before those molars come in, he cannot chew whole or even mashed food properly. Until then, food should be well pureed, or it can irritate the stomach.

When baby is old enough to discover his food differs from that of the rest of the family, it sometimes causes a struggle. He wants to eat what everyone else has. Remember, he doesn't have the discernment to realize it's hard for his stomach to handle unchewed, unpureed food. Resist the temptation to give in and allow him to eat what he wants. If he rejects food at one meal, don't become upset; merely wait until the next. Even the appetites of healthy babies may vary. After he's had mashed food, it is difficult to revert to puree. He will do it, though, when he learns that is all he'll get!

When old people lose their teeth they spend a lot of money to buy new ones. They don't just mash food up and swallow it—it makes them sick.

It's just like a country girl seeing electric lights—she's not going to want to wash lamp shades any more. Once a child has tasted mashed food from the table, he thinks he has to eat like his parents, but he can't digest it properly until he has something to chew it with. It comes out in the diaper as it goes in.

Convinced that it was better to delay giving table food, I tried various tactics to avoid a battle. Two things seemed particularly effective: feeding baby before the rest of the family eats and not giving him anything that would whet his appetite for table food—crackers, cookies, Cheerios.

Don't give your baby juice, carbonated drinks, or snacks between meals (see pages 158-159). Remember, meals need to be spaced 5-1/2 hours apart.

Children who eat between meals get potbellied, anemic, and sorry. Their stomachs never have a chance to empty, so they're always hungry but never hungry enough to eat a decent meal. A hog will eat a lot and stretch out to rest until it digests its food. Then it will eat some more. Even a hog's got enough sense to eat right. A cow, of course, has two stomachs so it can eat all day.

If children come to my clinic with potbellies and dry, thin hair, I always ask their mother if she feeds them between meals. If the mother says no, I check the soles of their shoes for crumbs. Finding any means there is probably snack food strewn all over the house. Eating between meals is so chaotic.

You see big potbellies on old people with the same eating patterns. They could be nice, neat people if they just ate three simple meals a day and stayed out of the doctor's office. [Eating sensibly could minimize the need for multiple doctor visits and prescriptions! Prescriptions should never be a substitute for healthful eating habits.]

The three major causes of tooth decay are eating between meals, carbonated drinks, and mouth breathing.

Weaning

Dr. Denmark stressed that infants need to be weaned at 7–8 months. By then they should be eating plenty of pureed food and taking sips of water from a cup. Most breast-fed babies never need a bottle and can be weaned directly to a cup (see pages 158-159). After weaning you don't need to add milk or formula to his diet. It can produce anemia. Milk also decreases his appetite for other vital foods (see pages 160-161).

Offer babies and children water at every meal but don't worry if they refuse, unless they are sick. Pureed foods contain a lot of water and your baby may not need to drink after eating. If your child is sick, refusing food, or the weather is especially hot, do carefully monitor his fluid intake (see Further Information on Preventing Dehydration, pages 76-78).

Sleep

When baby is trained to expect a consistent nap schedule, he'll usually be happy in bed even if he doesn't sleep the entire time. Remember to pull down the shades, close the door, and keep things as quiet as possible. Put a safe "friend" (doll, blanket, or toy animal) in with him at naptime and at night. It's good for him to be attached to a particular toy. Some children need less sleep and will wake up during naps or at night and play with it in the crib. That's fine and it enables you to do necessary household chores.

Morning is a better time for a nap. When baby sleeps in the morning and is awake all afternoon, he's tired and ready for bed shortly after supper.

Most children on a regular schedule won't object to staying in their cribs from 9:00 am to 12:00 noon. It's a routine that adds peace to the household.

If parents put their children to bed at a sensible hour, eventually they begin sleeping at the right time. Afternoon nappers are usually not good night sleepers. It's important for baby to go to bed early enough so mama and papa can have a break in the evening.

When I was a young, inexperienced doctor, a mother brought her two little daughters into my clinic and claimed it was impossible to get them to bed. She wanted me to prescribe a sedative for them.

I was puzzled and kept questioning her to determine the cause of her children's sleeplessness. Finally, I asked, "What time do they get up in the morning?"

"About 11:30," she responded.

"Well then, they shouldn't go to bed until 11:30 p.m.!" I told the mother. I advised her to get them up at 7 and give them breakfast. If she did that, they would be ready to go to bed at the right time.

Dr. Denmark's recommended morning nap schedule was invaluable to our family life. I followed it pretty strictly, so my babies came to expect it. Those three hours were precious, and I used them to accomplish any task that required concentration (paperwork, children's studies, important phone calls). I'm not sure I could have managed the home with any semblance of order if it were otherwise. I did encourage my little ones to stay up in the afternoon so they were definitely ready for bed by evening. I, too, was ready for them to go!

Two Years

A two-year old's the cutest thing there is. They say "I do," and they mean it. From two to six he is braver than he will ever be. He is brave enough to try anything, so that makes this period in his life a most important teaching period.[14]

Food, Schedules, Sleep

7:00 a.m.   Breakfast
12:30 p.m. Lunch
6:00 p.m.   Supper
            Bedtime

At 24 months, a child's appetite typically drops drastically. Growth slows, and he will begin eating about a fifth as much as before. The change is normal.

Continue serving him three meals a day and give him only water to drink. Fruit at meals is highly preferable to fruit juice. Again, make sure meals are spaced 5-1/2 hours apart for proper digestion and to help him develop more of an appetite.

Between 24 and 28 months (when baby has developed enough molars) is a good time to introduce table food. At this time he has the ability to grind his food properly.

Transitioning from "mush" to table food should take place gradually until the toddler is eating the same foods as the rest of the family. His need for fruit diminishes drastically. (Refer to Chapter 11, which details proper nutrition for the entire family.)

Typically, a two-year-old will want to major on starches and sweets. He wants bread, crackers, noodles, potatoes, and cookies. I would put vegetables and protein on my two-year-old's plate **first** when he was most hungry and not discourage him with big servings. After he had finished his vegetables and protein, he might have a starch. Desserts were kept out of sight except on special occasions and after he had eaten his other food. Don't be so concerned about the amounts of food, but about the type and quality of food he eats.

Avoid any snacks between meals! They will kill his already diminished appetite. Don't fight with him over food. (When my children are older, I do require them to eat certain things.) Mealtime should be a happy time. If he doesn't want to eat, calmly put the food away and wait for the next meal. He should be good and hungry by then!

At this age a child no longer needs a daytime nap and will sleep approximately twelve hours at night until he is six years old. Eliminating the naps will help him sleep earlier and better. Parents and older children can enjoy a quiet evening!

If mother elects to keep that daytime nap, she must expect baby to be more wakeful in the evenings and have a later bedtime. It is a choice she needs to make.

I encouraged my toddlers to have a "quiet time" in the morning when they were no longer napping. They usually sat down with books or toys. Quiet time for toddlers enables older home-schooled siblings to concentrate better on their studies and helps a younger, napping baby to sleep more soundly.

Sleep Disturbances

Sometimes a young child's sleep will be disturbed for no apparent reason. He may wake repeatedly, cry out, or grit his teeth. You need to look for the cause. Check for fever, congestion, bright lights and loud noises. To sleep well, infants must be positioned on their stomachs. A baby positioned on his back can easily wake himself up (See pages 16-19). Is your infant getting enough nourishment at his ten o'clock feeding? (See page 7)

Another common sleep disturbance is stinging alkaline urine which is often accompanied by a diaper rash. Don't give baby juice to drink. Juice and too much fruit can give him alkaline urine.

If your child has passed his second birthday and especially if he sucks fingers or thumbs, check for pinworms (see pages 69-70). Some children cannot settle down after overly rough play, especially if they have been tossed in the air.

Disturbing television images are a frequent culprit. Children are emotionally vulnerable and need their parents to protect them from confusing, emotionally tense, fast-paced, or frightening images. A child's free time should be spent playing outdoors, reading, or making things. What few programs they watch need to be wholesome and gentle (see Appendix II).

Bedtime is a great time for a song, story, and prayers. A little one who is ushered off to bed this way is much less likely to be troubled with nightmares.

Baby Schedule Summary
Birth to Three Months

6:00 a.m.   Feed (breast or bottle); sleep in open room.
9:30 a.m.   Bathe (as needed).
10:00 a.m. Feed (breast or bottle); nap and quiet time.
2:00 p.m.   Feed (breast or bottle); open room.
6:00 p.m.   Feed (breast or bottle); play time.
10:00 p.m. Feed (breast or bottle); check baby and put to bed
            for the night.

Three Months

Introduce solids at 10:00 a.m., 2:00 p.m., and 6:00 p.m.

6:00 a.m.   Feed.
9:30 a.m.   Bathe (as needed).
10:00 a.m. Feed; nap.
2:00 p.m.   Feed; playtime.
6:00 p.m.   Feed; put to bed.
10:00 p.m. Feed; put to bed for the night.

Four Months

Continue with milk and solids at all three meals.

7:00 a.m.   Feed.
9:00 a.m.   Bathe (as needed); put down for three-hour nap.
12:30 p.m. Feed; play time (no scheduled nap).
6:00 p.m.   Feed; put to bed (should sleep until morning).

Five Months

Continue four-month schedule. Add sips of water from a cup.

Seven Months to 24 Months

Continue four-month schedule. Wean baby from breast or formula (no need to add any milk to diet).

Two Years and Forward

Continue three meals daily. Transition to table food. No need for naps. Put to bed after supper.

Immunizations

The following are the vaccinations Dr. Denmark administered in her practice. She believed they are safe and vital to your child's health. They should be administered according to the following schedule:

Five months: DPT, polio
Six months: DPT, polio
Seven months: DPT, polio
Fifteen months: MMR

Note: DPT stands for diphtheria, pertussis, and tetanus. MMR stands for measles, mumps, and rubella. Pertusis is the whooping cough vaccine.

No additional vaccinations are necessary for a baby who doesn't go to day care. All babies should be examined for possible illness before having the vaccinations. Don't have a sick baby vaccinated. Vaccinations should be administered in the deltoid muscle of the arm. Massage the area well after administering.

The first shots shouldn't be given before five months because the baby's immune system hasn't developed enough to make sufficient antibodies. After the initial DPT's, he won't need a tetanus shot for ten years unless he receives a wound in a horse lot or from a gunshot or a rusty nail. For safety's sake, you may want to repeat the booster every ten years (see Vaccinations, Chapter Thirteen).

Occasionally a baby will develop fever from the vaccinations. It may begin four hours after the vaccination and last up to 24 hours. Aspirin (see pages 119-120) can be used to reduce the fever and help baby feel more comfortable. Dr. Denmark did not believe aspirin causes Reye's syndrome (See pages 72-73, 102-103).

Note: If an unvaccinated child contracts whooping cough and survives the disease without medication, he is immune for life. If he is cured with antibiotics, he is not immune and will need to be vaccinated to prevent further occurrence. Whooping cough is a serious illness and should always be treated with erythromycin (See Whooping Cough, pages 103-104, 109, 256-259; Ch. 13).

...this discovery we learned about immunization...the greatest lifesaver that has been found up to this time. Typhoid, tetanus, diphtheria, whooping cough, smallpox, polio, measles, pus-forming diseases, yellow fever, and many more diseases are rarely seen any more, for man has built in his own body, with the aid of small doses of the killer, an army [antibodies] that can protect him against the organisms that once caused sickness or death...[15]

You should say a word of thanks each day for immunizations and good drugs and for the blessing that your child does not have to suffer the long deadly illnesses your parents and grandparents had.[16]

Since the publishing of this book, one of the most common topics of discussion by readers has been that of vaccinations. Many parents are confused and alarmed by what they have read in news magazines or via the Internet.

Parents must make the best choices possible for their own child based on their own research. Bear in mind that Internet sources are often alarmist and inaccurate. Everything true and everything false can be found on the Internet. My husband and I are convinced that Dr. Denmark's recommendations are wise and believe that immunizations are a great blessing. However, there is no need to over vaccinate.

All of our children were vaccinated by Dr. Denmark except Jessica (born overseas) and our youngest, Emily. Dr. Denmark retired from practice not long after Emily was born. When Emily was an infant, we discovered first-hand the myriad of immunizations that are offered to new parents and something of the pressure exerted that they comply with CDC recommendations.

When offered vaccines for Emily, we tried to politely, calmly, and confidently inform the staff that we had done our own research and told them which shots we wanted and when. Most medical personnel are simply concerned for the health of the child and when reassured that parents are trying to act responsibly will not interfere.

We were informed at that time that DPT was now called Dtap and that the vaccination had been improved. After discovering that the vaccine had been altered, we opted to give her a fourth dose of Dtap instead of the three DPTs.

Occasionally, we will hear of a physician who is absolutely emphatic that each patient receive his dictated regimen of immunizations and that parents must follow every "jot and tittle" of his prescribed baby-care instructions. Some doctors have gone so far as to imply that those who do not follow their advice are guilty of negligence. New parents do not need this kind of intimidation. My suggestion is that parents find a physician who is not only competent medically, but has respect for parental authority and is flexible enough to allow parents to make some of their own decisions regarding care of their children.

Since the last edition of this book, we have learned the distressing information that many vaccines currently offered in the US were developed from aborted fetal tissue. When these vaccines were first developed, they probably came from sources which weren't morally objectionable. Those desiring to use the immunizations Dr. Denmark recommended could choose the alternate vaccines offered for DPT (Dtap: Diptheria, Tetanus, Pertussis) and polio. (see Appendix I). Currently, MMR has no alternate cell line offered in the United States. As important a vaccination as MMR is, my husband and I could not support using it. Our prayer is that in the future it can be obtained from other sources.

We treat babies more like toys, but they're human beings. When you bring a baby into the world, he is your responsibility. That child's not supposed to make you feel big; you're supposed to make him feel big. You need to give that child a chance.

Notes

1. Leila Daughtry-Denmark, MD, *Every Child Should Have a Chance* (Atlanta, GA: 1971), 15

2. Denmark, *Every Child Should Have a Chance*, 13

3. Denmark, 41

4. Denmark, 17

5. Denmark, 16

6. Denmark, 16

7. Denmark, 17

8. Denmark, 5

9. Denmark, 14

10. Denmark, 3

11. Denmark, 4

12. Denmark, 78

13. Denmark, 83

14. Denmark, 25

15. Denmark, 136

16. Denmark, 40

ℰ 2 ℭ
Danger Signs Indicating Emergency

It's 2:30 a.m. A frantic young mother picks up the phone and dials, cuddling a four-month-old infant in her left arm. A sleepy voice answers, "Hello...Dr. Denmark."

"Dr. Denmark, this is Madia Bowman."

"Yes, I hope everything is all right at the Bowman house."

"I apologize for calling you at this hour, but I didn't know what to do. My baby has a terribly high fever! I just took her temperature rectally and the thermometer says 100°."

One might guess that baby Malinda survived the night! Under Dr. Denmark's patient instruction, I eventually learned to distinguish a true emergency from an illness that can wait until morning for professional attention. Children are seldom sick at convenient times. It's usually after office hours that a fever rises or a stomachache becomes severe. The following guidelines can help you distinguish true emergencies.

Fever

If a child has a fever, its probably due to a common illness. However, it's a good idea to check him for meningitis.

Procedure

1. Lay him on his back.
2. Put a hand under the back of his neck and bend his head forward gently, bringing the chin toward the chest. A fussy child may stiffen his neck to resist examination, so calm and distract him while you check. **If the neck is stiff and will not bend, take him to the hospital emergency room.**
3. Lay the child on his back.
4. Lift his knee and try to raise the leg at a right angle from body.

   If legs are very stiff, it also indicates an emergency. A bulging fontanel (soft spot) on a newborn may also indicate meningitis (See page 263-264).

Abdominal Pain

If a child has stomach pain, first determine whether he has swallowed anything unusual. If he has, call your local poison control center immediately and follow their instructions. If he hasn't swallowed anything requiring a medical emergency, check him for appendicitis.

Procedure

1. Lay the child on his back.
2. Distract him with a toy.
3. Press his stomach between the right hipbone and navel
4. If he experiences sharp pain, he'll react to pressure in an obvious way. Sharp pain in this region indicates acute appendicitis. **Take him immediately to the emergency room and do not give him an enema.**

Note: Don't ask the child if this or that hurts. Children will normally answer "yes" whether they feel pain or not. It's important to distract him while pressing his abdomen.

Other Signs of Emergency

- Seizure
- A lot of red blood from rectum
- Severe respiratory difficulty
- Cyanosis (turning purple or blue indicates heart problems)

Dr. Denmark recommended training in CPR techniques and relief of airway obstruction (choking). Contact your local hospital for classes offered in your community. It's a good idea to post the telephone number to your local poison control center in a convenient place. We have found them to be helpful and often reassuring when our children have breathed, touched, or consumed anything that causes concern.

Don't fail to call 911 if your child's life is in imminent danger. If necessary, it's best to go directly to a hospital whose emergency room specializes in the care of children.

If a mother doesn't have a good idea about what's wrong with her child, she shouldn't mess around and wait until he's in bad trouble. Most any doctor can recognize an emergency. In an emergency you need to go directly to where they can handle it.

ঙ 3 ८ঙ
Common Ailments

"Ow, ow! Mommy, I have a terrible cut on my finger!"
"David, come here and let me see your hand. Where is it?"
"On this one. Ow, it hurts!"
"I don't see it. Show me where the cut is."
"Well…maybe it's on the other hand."

Soothing small hurts, real or imaginary, is an ordinary part of a mother's day. Cuts, scrapes, burns, bee stings—the list seems endless. In my early days of mothering, I was dialing Dr. Denmark for all kinds of minor complaints. As my family grew, so did the frequency of the phone calls. It finally occurred to me that I was repeating the same questions.

Cataloging her recommended treatment was helpful to me and a time-saver for Dr. Denmark. **Refer to Chapter 9 for information on recommended medications.**

Stomachache

First, check the child for possible poisoning or appendicitis (See pages 48-49). If that's ruled out, watch for other symptoms—gas, diarrhea, vomiting, fever. With diarrhea or vomiting, he may have an intestinal infection or salmonella (food poisoning). Enemas are highly effective in combating intestinal disorders (see chapter four). If the stomachache is accompanied by a fever, he may need antibiotics (see chapter seven). For intestinal gas, a dose of milk of magnesia* followed by a drink of warm water often brings relief. If an adult is ill, it might be helpful to drink water as hot as people usually drink tea or coffee. Children will not want to drink it as hot as adults.

Dosage for Milk of Magnesia*

0–6 months: 1/2 teaspoon
6 months–6 years: One teaspoon
6 years–adult: Two teaspoons

Should the pain continue, check periodically for appendicitis and consult a physician.

Stomachs are very sensitive and are designed by the Creator to vomit easily as a form of protection against poison and bacteria. If a child has frequent stomachaches, observe him carefully over a period of time. Investigate the kinds of food he eats, eating patterns, the time of day stomachaches occur, and the environment and emotional state of the child. Sometimes children complain of stomachaches in an effort to gain attention. You may have to "play detective" to discover the cause.

Emergency Situations Related to Abdominal Pain: appendicitis (See pages 48-49), severe pain accompanied by bloody stools and/or a lot of red blood from the anus.

Motion Sickness

Motion sickness is more common in some families than in others. The tendency depends on the structure of the inner ear. It may be treated with Dramamine*.

We discovered early on that Susanna has a tendency to have motion sickness. Our family went camping when she was an infant. Everyone seemed healthy and excited as we pulled out of the driveway. Later our 15-passenger van began winding around mountain roads and poor Susanna became progressively more fretful.

I've always been a "good sailor," so the possibility of motion sickness did not occur to me until we arrived at the campsite. I assumed we had brought a stomach bug to Vogel State Park! After we set up camp and her world stopped spinning, the nausea subsided and Susanna's cheerful little smiles reappeared. Now, years later, she always gets a dose of Dramamine before long trips. It makes her sleepy, but much more comfortable.

Headaches

Headaches often accompany colds, respiratory infections, flu, food poisoning, and fatigue. If a young child complains of his eyes hurting, it could indicate that he has a headache.

Menstruation, excitement, eye strain, allergies, and too much sodium are also common causes for teenagers' headaches. A child learning to read could be straining his eyes by reading too long and/or might need glasses. Gatorade, potato chips, and other salty foods should be avoided, and an eye exam may be in order.

Migraine headaches seem to run in families and can be stimulated by allergies due to almost anything. Some children have migraines after smelling asphalt, some after eating an onion. The child should be studied to see if there is a pattern to the headaches.

Sometimes, the cause of headaches is difficult to determine. If they are frequent and seem to continue for no explainable reason, take your child for a physical examination. If the exam doesn't pinpoint the cause, he may need more extensive testing (MTR, CT scans) to rule out the possibility of a tumor.

Treatment for common headache: aspirin* and a drink of warm water.

Skin

Cuts

Wide or deep cuts need immediate stitching at a doctor's office before infection sets in. Wash minor cuts with soap and warm water. Rinse thoroughly and cleanse with alcohol. Thoroughly cleansing wounds with an antiseptic is important to promote healing and prevent possible blood poisoning (septicemia).

Silvadene cream* can be applied after cleansing to prevent or treat infection. Do not use peroxide. Most small cuts can be covered loosely with a bandaid to keep them clean. If the cut is open, tape it closed securely with medical adhesive or steri strips. Do not wet or otherwise disturb the taped cut for seven days.

Scrapes and Scratches

Clean a scrape or scratch the same way you treat a cut. Apply no dressing and keep it as dry as possible.

A Hard-to-Heal Scrape

When my son David was five years old, he scraped the inside of his ankle. The abrasion wasn't large, but he constantly rubbed it with his shoe and knocked it open. If he didn't wear shoes, dirt got into the wound. If I put on a Band-Aid, it became moist and oozed (typical of scrapes).

After a week, the scrape began to look worse. The area around it was turning red, indicating infection. Out of desperation, I forbade him to go outside, hoping to keep the scrape clean. He promptly tripped over a toy and set it bleeding again. I cleaned him up, confined him to a chair and called Dr. Denmark. Following her instructions, I covered the scrape with a generous application of Silvadene* and a gauze bandage adhesive taped to his ankle. I changed the bandage at least once a day or whenever it got dirty. It was quite a trick to give him a bath without wetting the ankle. The treatment worked wonders, and the scrape healed quickly. I was thankful I didn't have to straitjacket my bouncy five-year-old to enable his ankle to heal!

Severe Infection

Possible Symptoms

- A lot of redness around the wound
- Fever
- A knot in the groin (leg or foot wound)
- A knot in the armpit (arm or hand wound)
- A red streak

Treatment

1. Apply Silvadene cream* generously.
2. Cover with a gauze bandage.
3. Change the dressing daily.
4. Keep the wound from getting wet.
5. Give antibiotics to fight infection. Ampicillin or penicillin* are good options.
6. You may have to consult a doctor.

Burns

A third-degree burn is a deep, severe burn. Skin may be burned away, and some flesh will be charred. Do not try to care for this kind of wound yourself. Take the child immediately to the hospital to be treated.

First- and second-degree burns cause redness and tenderness, and the skin might blister.

Treatment

1. Wipe the burned skin at once with bleach*.
2. Immediately rinse gently but **thoroughly** with water.
3. Pat gently with sterile cotton.
4. Keep the affected area clean and dry. If there is any break in the skin, continue treatment by:
5. Put Silvadene cream* on gauze thickly.
6. Place dressing over burn.
7. Bind by wrapping with more gauze.
8. Leave dressing on for four days.
9. Redress after four days if necessary.
10. Keep the affected area dry.

Note: Should the burn become soiled after the initial treatment, clean with alcohol. When blisters drain on their own, wipe with alcohol and apply Silvadene cream*.

Note: Dr. Jefferson Flowers (See page 132) recommends soaking minor burns in cold water for twenty minutes before applying medicine.

Eczema

If a child's skin is scaly, often in patches, he may have eczema, which tends to break out where the most perspiration occurs. Eczema is an allergic reaction to some environmental factor. Any irritant can cause eczema if allergy is present. In addition to treating the condition, try to play "detective" and determine the cause of the allergy. Common offenders are food, soap, fabrics, and tobacco smoke (See pages 11, 29, 113-115). If your child is prone to eczema, carefully rinse away soap and shampoo when bathing him. If a baby has eczema, bathe him only once a week, rinsing thoroughly. Avoid perfumed soaps and those that leave a residue. Ivory is often the best. Every individual's skin is different, so keep trying various soaps until you find one that seems to work well with your child's skin.

Treatment

If the eczema is merely scaly,

1. Wash skin with sterile water and dry.
2. Apply one 0.1% Kenalog cream* twice a day.

If the eczema looks infected (like an ulcer),

1. Wash with sterile water and dry.
2. Apply Silvadene cream* twice a day, alternating with the Kenalog cream.* For example, Silvadene in the morning; Kenalog at noon; Silvadene in the evening, Kenalog at bedtime.

If the eczema involves a fungal infection (characterized by watery, scaly skin),

1. Apply Silvadene cream twice a day.
2. Shake nystatin powder* on top of the Silvadene.

Note: Kenalog cream* is a steroid and should only be used for short-term treatment.

Rashes (General)

There are a host of reasons an individual breaks out in a rash. Generally speaking, but not always, the following principles apply: A systemic rash covers the entire body or is concentrated in areas of heavier perspiration such as the crook of the arms or back of the knees. It is a reaction to something the child has eaten or drunk. A rash which covers only parts of the body and isn't concentrated in those areas is a reaction to something contacted by the skin such as new-fabric dye, poison ivy, or soaps.

A simple test may enable you to determine if a rash is caused by an allergy. Scratch your child's skin with moderate friction (do not break the skin or inflict pain!). Closely observe the skin's reaction to the scratch. If it welts up and/or becomes very red, then there is likely extra histamine in the skin. This indicates your child's rash is probably allergy-related. If the skin does not react this way to scratching, then look for other causes such as: insect bites, infection, chicken pox, measles, or scarlet fever.

If your child has a rash as a reaction to a particular food, give him a dose of milk of magnesia* to help cleanse his digestive tract. If his skin is reacting to something topical such as new-fabric dye (See page 113) wipe the affected area with alcohol to get the dye off and wash the garment. Chlor-Trimeton (or Benadryl) syrup* can help reduce itching. With any severe rash or one associated with a fever, call your physician.

Poison Ivy or Poison Oak

The rash is characterized by redness and blisters and is caused by contact with the oil from the plant. It will last 14 days from the time of contact.

Treatment (same treatment for jellyfish stings)

1. Keep the affected area completely dry to prevent infection.
2. Chlor-Trimeton or Benadryl syrup* will reduce itching.
3. Caladryl*, calamine* or witch hazel applied locally also reduces itching.

If your child has previously exhibited a sensitivity to poison ivy and has recently been exposed, the following procedure removes the oil and may minimize allergic reaction. It must be done before redness and swelling develop.

1. Rub the exposed skin at once with bleach.
2. Rinse with water immediately and **thoroughly**.

If the child's skin has already developed an allergic reaction, the same procedure may be followed with diluted bleach* (one tablespoon bleach mixed with one quart water). Blisters develop as the skin attempts to shed the poisonous ivy oil. **Even if blisters become exceptionally large, don't attempt to drain them.** Dab them with alcohol after they drain on their own, and apply Silvadene cream*. Silvadene may also be applied if the skin becomes infected (twice daily).

Our Steven is highly allergic to poison ivy. The first time he was exposed, his little face swelled up to where it was barely recognizable. I remember watching him stare into the bathroom mirror. "Am I still Steven?" was his pathetic question.

David, who has no problem with the ivy, took advantage of Steven's handicap. He would badger his big brother mercilessly and then run into the poison ivy patch where he could not be followed. "Hey Steven, come get me!"

One afternoon Steven had enough. He ploughed into the poison ivy, grabbed his brother, and then raced to the kitchen for a bleach rinse. Retribution at last!

Athlete's Foot

Athlete's foot is a fungal infection characterized by an itchy rash on the soles of the feet and between the toes. It can cause the skin to crack and peel.

Treatment

1. Wash feet with bleach* water (1 tablespoon in 1 qt. water).
2. Rinse immediately and **thoroughly** with water.
3. Keep feet clean and dry, and wear cotton socks with tennis shoes.
4. Apply nystatin topical powder* twice daily until infection heals.

Note: Repeat washing once a day until it heals.

Ringworm

Ringworm is not caused by a worm but is a fungal infection most often found on children who lack a balanced diet. It is a round, itchy rash with a red-edged ring which temporarily destroys the hair on location. The rash usually consists of one or two patches the size of a quarter or larger. These can occur anywhere on the body.

Ringworm should be treated with an antifungal medication such as nystatin topical powder* twice a day until it disappears. Examine the child's diet to see if there is a deficiency, especially in vitamin B (see Chapter Eleven).

Impetigo

Impetigo is a staph infection of the skin. It usually looks like a burn and may have a greenish color. It can develop from anything that causes a break in the skin—a bite, burn, sunburn, nettle, or cut. The skin peels.

Treatment
1. Soak off the scabs gently in warm water.
2. Wash the area well with soap and water. Be sure to rinse off all the soap, and don't make the area bleed.
3. Dab on Silvadene cream*.

The procedure may need to be repeated twice a day for up to one week.

Sunburn

A child needs a moderate amount of sunshine for good health. The vitamin D obtained from the sun is vital, but don't allow him to bake in the sun. Since the use of sunscreens is questionable, it's best to cover the skin with clothing. If he plays a long time in the sun he needs a hat to guard against sunstroke as well as sunburn. A kimono is ideal for babies playing in the sand.

Treatment
1. The child's skin may be bathed gently.
2. Wipe the burn with witch hazel or alcohol and keep the skin clean.
3. If there is a break in the skin, Silvadene cream* should be applied twice daily until it heals.

Boils

With a true abscess, there is a white (not clear) blister on top.

Treatment
1. Clean with alcohol.
2. Use sterilized needle to open boil.
3. Pull skin away from center to drain (don't mash in).
4. After draining, dress with Silvadene cream*.

Applying hot compresses or soaking boils in warm water will make them feel better. To make a compress, dip a clean soft cloth in hot water, squeeze it out and apply it to the affected area. If there is a great deal of heat or redness around the boil and/or a red streak appears, seek professional help at once.

Chapped Skin

As soon as the weather turns chilly, my children get chapped hands and faces. The skin on the back of the boys' hands used to resemble sandpaper.

Dr. Denmark recommended a very light layer of Vaseline (petroleum jelly) applied to chapped skin twice a day. Instruct your children to rinse soap thoroughly and carefully dry their hands. Discourage them from licking their lips.

Blisters (friction)

Blisters can be caused by many different things (see Blisters in Index). One way they commonly form is when the skin is rubbed repeatedly by a hard surface (new shoes, tennis racket, shovel, etc.).

Treatment
1. Try to eliminate—or cushion the skin from—the source of friction.
2. Keep the blister clean and undisturbed.
3. After it drains on its own, wipe it with alcohol and apply Silvadene cream* twice daily until it heals.
4. Try to keep the drained blister clean and dry.

Bites and Stings

Bee, Wasp, Fire Ant

Treatment

1. Promptly apply bleach*. Must apply before swelling and redness occur.
2. Wash off immediately and **thoroughly** with water.
3. Apply witch hazel or alcohol.
4. Give dose of Chlor-Trimeton or Benadryl syrup* every eight hours if needed.
5. Can apply Caladryl* or calamine lotion* to reduce itching.

Dosage for Chlor-Trimeton*

0-6 months: 1/2 teaspoon syrup or 1/4 of a 4 mg tablet crushed

6 months-adult: One teaspoon syrup or 1/2 of a 4 mg tablet crushed

(Normally administered every 8 hours as needed.)

For any severe allergic reaction evidenced by breathing difficulties or welts covering the body, take the child to the emergency room.

Ticks

Treatment

1. Apply gasoline to the tick with a Q-Tip. Be careful not to touch the surrounding skin. Kerosene and Raid are also effective.
2. After one minute, pull the tick off with tweezers. Be careful to remove the entire tick, including the head.
3. Wash well with soap and water.
4. Apply Mercurochrome* or alcohol to cleanse the area.

Mosquito and Other Common Insect Bites

Treatment

Wipe bites with alcohol or Mercurochrome*. If an allergic reaction occurs, resulting in large welts, give the child Chlor-Trimeton or Benadryl syrup* in the same dosage as for bee stings. Itching can be treated with Caladryl*, calamine lotion* or witch hazel.

Scratched bites can become infected with impetigo and begin to ooze. If this happens, treat with Silvadene cream* twice a day.

Note: Any bites that blister should be cleansed again after the blisters drain on their own. Dab with alcohol or Mercurochrome* to cleanse and apply Silvadene cream* afterward.

Minor Dog and Cat Bites

Treatment

Cleanse the wound thoroughly with soap and water, then alcohol. Leave it open to the air. Study the animal to be sure its behavior is normal. Observe it for possible illness. Inquire as to whether it has received its shots. If the animal is ill, call a physician and animal control immediately. If your child has been bitten and you cannot find the animal, consult a physician immediately.

Note: It's also a good idea to carefully clean animal scratches to prevent infection.

Venomous Snake Bites

Treatment

Give the child two teaspoons of Chlor-Trimeton or Benadryl syrup* (one 4mg tablet), put ice directly on the puncture wounds, and go immediately to the hospital emergency room.

Lice

Lice are recognized by severe itching and small white specks attached to the hair that cannot be easily removed. The specks (eggs) are usually around the ears. Use Kwell* and follow the directions on the box. Special fine-tooth combs help remove the eggs and can be found at most pharmacies.

Swallowing Objects

If a child swallows a medium-sized object such as a marble, coin, or pin, look for it in his stools for up to ten days. If the object is not passed or he is experiencing pain, consult a physician. An X-ray may be necessary.

Blow to the Head

Elevate the head and try to keep the child as quiet as possible to minimize internal bleeding. I have used suckers to console a child who received one. Vomiting is common with head injuries and may not be a danger sign. Apply ice to the bump if it doesn't make the child cry.

Look for danger signs—eyes not focusing, unequal dilation in the pupils, poor sense of balance, or other abnormal behavior. Shining a flashlight in the child's pupils and observing the response of his pupils will help detect unequal dilation. If such signs are present, go to the hospital emergency room.

A blow to the side of the head is potentially more dangerous than on the front or back because the skull is thinner on the side. Heavier bones over the eyes and at the back protect the brain better.

Conjunctivitis

Conjunctivitis is caused by clogged tear ducts, often induced by allergies and colds. Pus develops in the eyes when the ducts get stopped up. If not treated, they may become red and infected. Many call this condition "pinkeye," although it is not true "pink-eye."

Treatment

Opening tear duct:

1. Place a small piece of sterile cotton on your index finger.
2. Put your finger under the child's eye. Gently press the corner next to the nose and pull down.
3. Repeat the procedure four times daily.

Warm compresses:

1. Take a warm wet washcloth or ball of cotton and squeeze it out, placing it over the eye for a few minutes.
2. When the compress cools, dip it in warm water and repeat the procedure.
3. Soak the eye in this manner four times daily.

If the eye does not respond to the treatment after a few days or the eyeball becomes red, see a doctor.

Dr. Denmark used Argyrol* for years to treat eye infections. She put one drop in each eye daily for three days (never longer).

Occasionally a child is born with a closed tear duct that must be opened surgically. Surgery may be necessary if the eye continues to secrete pus following full treatment.

Fainting

Turn the child on his stomach and wait for him to revive. If he doesn't revive immediately, hold some ammonia under his nose for a few seconds and cover his face with a cold cloth. If this procedure does not revive him, go immediately to the emergency room. In any case consult a physician to determine the cause for his fainting.

Menstrual Pain

Menstrual pain is caused by the tightening of the cervical muscle during menses.

Anything which makes a young girl tense can aggravate menstrual pain. Encourage her to relax so blood can flow easily through the cervix.

Treatment

1. Avoid all caffeine.
2. Drink a glass of hot water and take an aspirin*.
3. Stretch out on the bed on her stomach and rest.

Minor Mouth Sores

If a child gets mouth sores frequently, study his diet for a possible deficiency that would lower the body's resistance. Lack of vitamin B is a common one.

Treatment

Paint the sores with a little Mercurochrome* on the end of a Q-Tip once a day for three days. Gargling with Listerine* or salt water may be helpful. The salt content should be no more than one teaspoon per quart of water. A higher concentration may irritate the tissues of the mouth and throat.

Swimmer's Ear

Putting one's head under water can cause infection. If your child complains of an earache after swimming, press the V-shaped protrusion on the outside part of his ear above the earlobe next to his cheek. If the pressure is painful, he may have swimmer's ear. An abscessed ear does not hurt more when pressed (See pages 94-96). Swimmer's ear is a fungal infection and will need ear drops prescribed by a physician. Use until the pain goes away.

A few drops of rubbing alcohol in the ear canal right after swimming will help remove the water that promotes the infection. The alcohol lowers the surface tension of the water, enabling it to run out easily. You may dry the ear canal with a towel afterward.

Swimming pools are about the dirtiest things we have created. There are urine and feces in pools. They're filthy…but it is important for children to learn to swim.

Our ears are similar to those of a dog, cat, or horse. You never see any of them put their heads under water when they're swimming. They have too much sense.

I was born and reared near Savannah, Georgia, but we lived on a farm so I never learned to swim as a child. As an adult I had nightmares about kids drowning. The dreams repeated the same scenario —there were children stranded on a sand bar. The tide was coming in, and I was helpless to do anything.

At age 61, I became determined to learn to swim. We were traveling on a ship at the time, and there was a pool available to the passengers. I borrowed Mary's bathing suit (Eustace thought I had lost my mind), got up early to avoid being seen, and began to teach myself. There were a few kids up at that early hour, and they tried to coach me. "Dr. Denmark, if you don't put your head under the water, you'll never learn to swim," they'd say.

"Never will my head get wet," I told them. Ten days later, oof, oof, I was going the length of the pool! My head never went under, but I learned to swim and the nightmares stopped.

Nosebleeds

Nosebleeds occur when the septum vessels are broken. They are close to the surface and rupture if the nose is twisted or bumped. Nosebleeds are more common in some families than others.

Treatment

1. Have the child stand up straight. Don't lift his chin.
2. Put pressure under the child's nose by pressing down on the upper lip, and put an ice pack on the nose.
3. In a few minutes a clot will have formed, and the bleeding stops. The clot can then be gently blown out. If nosebleeds occur frequently be sure to consult a doctor. The nose may have to be cauterized. If they still continue, the child's blood should be studied for possible leukemia, rheumatic fever, or diabetes.

Pinworms

Pinworms are everywhere. A child can contract them by eating with unwashed hands, biting nails, sucking fingers, and eating mucous from his nose. Symptoms are restless sleep, gritting teeth, and crying out while sleeping. Observe the child's anus with a flashlight at night in the dark. The white, thin worms are often evident. They are twice as long as an eyelash and pointed on the ends.

Treatment

1. One Vermox* tablet a day for three days. Dosage is the same for all ages.
2. Disinfect door knobs and toilet handles by wiping them with rubbing alcohol.

A child can get pinworms repeatedly as long as he puts his hands in his mouth. Treat him each time, but he should not have Vermox more frequently than every three months.

Note: Many physicians prescribe one tablet of Vermox, one time for pinworms. Others prescribe two dosages a week apart. There are also over the counter medications available to parents. Dr. Denmark, however, believed the preceding treatment to be most effective.

Styes

A stye is a small boil formed on the rim of an eyelid.

Treatment

Apply warm compresses two or three times daily. Compresses may be made by dipping a clean soft cloth or ball of cotton in warm water, squeezing it out, and applying it to the affected area. After the boil begins to drain on its own, apply Silvadene cream* twice a day until complete healing takes place.

*For information on recommended medications and substances refer to the following pages:

Medication	Page	Medication	Page
Argyrol	125	Kenelog cream	126
Ampicillin	125, Ch 7	Kwell	123
Aspirin	119-120	Listerine	123
Auralgan	125-126	Macrodantin	126
Benadryl	121	Mercurochrome	123
Bleach	127	Milk of magnesia	124
Caladryl lotion	121	Nystatin powder	126
Calamine lotion	121	Pedialyte	124
Clor-Trimeton	121	Penicillin	125, Ch 7
Dramamine	122	Silvadene cream	126
Erythromycin	125, Ch 7	Vermox	127

✌ 4 ✍
Digestive Disorders and Enemas

It was a beautiful morning, and things were running smoothly for the Bowman household. The older children were seated at the breakfast table. Baby David was gobbling down a huge bowl of mush. I had just wiped his hands and face when his entire breakfast came up all over the highchair tray.

He couldn't be sick, I thought. He must have just gagged. I'll watch him and see. When the mess was cleaned up, I placed another bowl of mush on the tray and began spooning it into his mouth. Suddenly, I heard telltale noises from three-year-old Esther. She had vomited on the table and the floor as well.

With a sense of desperation, I grabbed a rag and several towels. The telephone rang. After hoisting a crying baby David onto my hip, I answered—wrong number. No sooner had I put down the phone when David threw up his second breakfast onto my shoulder. A minute later, Esther was sick again, this time on the living room couch.

I made a beeline for the milk of magnesia and took the enema bag out of the closet. Whew! What a way to start the day!

Diagnosing Digestive Disorders

When a child has stomach pain he should first be checked for possible poisoning or appendicitis (See pages 48-49). If the stomach pain is mild, a dose of milk of magnesia may be all he needs (See pages 51-52). Dr. Denmark recommended milk of magnesia for a variety of intestinal ailments. Its laxative effect helps the digestive tract recover.

On Dr. Denmark's recommended diet, constipation shouldn't be a problem, but if it occurs, milk of magnesia is again recommended. When a child's stools are slightly abnormal (unusual consistency and strong odor) or he has mild diarrhea, give him milk of magnesia and watch for other symptoms. A fever may indicate the need for an antibiotic (See page 80). With vomiting and persistent diarrhea, enemas are probably in order.

Purpose of Enemas

Vomiting and diarrhea are immediate signals that the body is trying to cleanse itself of bacteria or food poisoning. Giving medication merely to stop the symptoms is not a wise method of treating intestinal disorders. The foreign matter needs to be expelled to enable the body to recover quickly.

In most cases, enemas are particularly effective in treating digestive disorders. They help stop vomiting and diarrhea, prevent dehydration, and are an effective guard against **Reye's syndrome.** Reye's syndrome is caused by vomiting and diarrhea after which the blood becomes so thick it clots (vascular coagulation). Enemas can prevent thickening of the blood. If a child cannot keep down fluid and has diarrhea, enemas prevent dehydration because fluid is absorbed through the colon. The chemical makeup of Dr. Denmark's enemas soothes the stomach and restores the balance of electrolytes. Enemas can also help bring down a high fever by replenishing vital body fluids.

I frequently saw Reye's syndrome when I worked in the slums. Children would come in so dehydrated they looked like mummies. I remember one particular case when I was interning at Egleston Hospital. Dr. Hoppy said to me, "Dr. Denmark, there's no point in trying to treat that child. It's simply too late." I put a needle in the child's arm and pumped in 50 ccs of 50 percent glucose. The baby was playing in a few minutes. He wasn't dehydrated anymore. The first thing a doctor will do for a person with Reye's syndrome is to put him on IV's in an effort to dilute the blood and keep it from clotting. If the blood clots, the patient will die or become brain damaged [See pages 102-103].

Standard Enema
Method
1. Purchase Enema bag kit (See pages 122-123).
2. Give child milk of magnesia orally (dosage indicated below).
3. Wait two hours.
4. Administer standard enema.

Milk of Magnesia Dosage (see page 124)
0–6 months: 1/2 teaspoon
6 months–6 years: One teaspoon
6 years–adult: Two teaspoons

If the child vomits the milk of magnesia within ten minutes, repeat the dose once and then don't give him anything else until it's time for the enema. The standard enema consists of boiled water cooled to body temperature and mixed with baking soda.

Measurements for Enema Solution
0–1 year: 1/4 teaspoon baking soda and 8 oz. water
1 year–6 years: One teaspoon baking soda and 1 pint water
6 years–adult: Two teaspoons baking soda and quart of water

Procedure

1. Hang solution-filled enema bag.
2. Expel air from tube by letting a little water flow from nozzle (or pipe). Pinch off tube quickly to prevent wasting the rest of the solution.
3. Put Vaseline (petroleum jelly) on appropriate size nozzle.
4. Sit down, spread a towel over your lap, and lay your child (tummy down) over the towel. Carefully insert nozzle 1 to 1-1/2 inches into rectum, with tip pointing toward his navel. It is often helpful to twist the nozzle a little as it is inserted in order to get past the sphincter muscles.
5. Hold buttocks, release the solution, and let it go in slowly.
6. It's best not to let the solution be expelled for ten minutes. Hold the baby's buttocks together to prevent early expulsion.
7. After ten minutes I often double diapered my infants and put them in their crib to contain messes (a cloth diaper and diaper cover over a disposable).

Note: With younger children I have hung the enema bag on a shower curtain rod and sat on a closed toilet seat next to the shower. Children old enough to self-administer the enema can stand in the shower and hang the enema bag from the shower head. Remind an older child to angle the nozzle towards his navel, release the solution, and wait until it has all gone in. Also remind him to hold it for ten minutes if possible before using the toilet. Nauseous children can be very dizzy, so carefully monitor the situation. I usually stand outside the bathroom door until they are finished.

The sooner the enema is administered, the more effective it is in cleansing the digestive tract of offending food or bacteria because there has been less time for absorption. Start with the milk of magnesia right after your child first vomits, and two hours later administer the enema (if the child is still sick and needs it). Occasionally a hard stool will block fluid. Administer the enema gently without forcing. Sometimes, sliding nozzle slightly in and out of the rectum a few times will better allow water to flow.

With excessive vomiting and diarrhea, the body may absorb most or all of the enema instead of discharging it. Absorption pre-vents dehydration. When a child is given an enema, he may expel the solution up to 12 hours later in the form of watery stools. If he is still having frequent, watery stools after 12 hours, they should be attributed to diarrhea, not the enema.

Enemas should be followed with a gentle diet. (See pages 78-79)

Retention Enema (Tea Enema)

If the child continues to vomit and cannot retain fluids after you have given a standard enema, a retention enema may be indi-cated to prevent dehydration and restore the balance of electrolytes.

Measurements for Enema Solution

1. Put 1 individual-sized tea bag (plain black tea) in 10 oz. water. Boil 3 minutes. Stir the tea bag around in the water and remove.
2. Mix the following:
    *   8 oz. tea solution
    *   24 oz. boiled water
    *   1/2 teaspoon baking soda
    *   1/2 teaspoon salt
    *   2 tablespoons dextrose or white Karo syrup (light corn syrup)

Procedure

Use the same basic procedure as for the standard enema (refer page 74) only with small, multiple doses. Warm the above mixture to body temperature and give 8 oz. as an enema every two hours, for four doses.

For example:

- 8 oz. at 10:00 a.m.
- 8 oz. at 12:00 noon
- 8 oz. at 2:00 p.m.
- 8 oz. at 4:00 p.m.

All ages have the same dosage—even infants. It's best if the enema solutions are retained for ten minutes before expulsion.

There is no question in my mind that enemas have saved us dozens of trips to the emergency room. Several of my children seem to have particularly sensitive stomachs. When they start vomiting, nothing stays down. It can be pretty dangerous and scary, especially with an infant. With severe vomiting, I resort to the retention enema and it works wonders. Usually by the second dose, vomiting has stopped.

Some doctors would lose their false teeth if they heard my advice about enemas—but enemas certainly do work!

One doctor told me, "Enemas went out with the Greeks!" Not so. My patients use them with great success. And I've never had a child develop Reye's syndrome who was treated with enemas.

Further Information on Preventing Dehydration

Dehydration is of concern when a child cannot retain fluids over an extended period of time because of severe vomiting and/or diarrhea. It can be life threatening. Symptoms are sunken eyes, rapid heart beat, lack of urination, and general weakness.

If your child is thirsty, give him water even if he vomits it up. His body will absorb some of it. Make sure the water is warm. Pedialyte can be given along with the enema to restore the electrolyte balance in a child who has had digestive problems. It is helpful for any age.

If you are concerned that your infant is becoming dehydrated, give him an enema and offer him frequent drinks of Pedialyte and warm water. Don't nurse or bottle feed more frequently than the recommended schedule (See page 42). Increasing the frequency of "milk meals" may further irritate his stomach and be counterproductive.

A Lesson Learned

One of our daughters was 18 months old when the following incident occurred. She had been very chipper, but her bowels were not normal. We had changed one or two bad diapers a day for close to a week. Her stools were of abnormal consistency with an unusually strong odor. She had no fever or vomiting, so I merely gave her some milk of magnesia and watched her behavior.

Suddenly baby's appetite dropped, but there were still no other symptoms. We speculated that the muggy weather might be affecting her.

For two days she ate very little, and I was becoming concerned. The evening of the second day I again dosed her with a little milk of magnesia and put her to bed. My plan was to give her an enema in the morning and call Dr. Denmark if her appetite didn't improve. That night she seemed restless and weak. I chided myself for being overly concerned. Surely she was just tired. I was pushing the alarm button for no good reason. Hadn't I done that numerous times in the past?

At 5:00 a.m. I awoke and checked her. To my dismay, I found her so weak she could hardly sit. I immediately called Dr. Denmark. She asked me some questions, and I checked her pulse rate. Dr. Denmark concluded that our baby had been fighting a relatively mild intestinal infection but was in serious condition because of dehydration.

I quickly gave her a retention enema and frequent sips of Pedialyte or warm water to restore her electrolyte balance and fluids. She regained strength and later her appetite.

In retrospect I was baffled. How in the world had she become dehydrated? I had always been careful to watch my babies' fluid intake and retention, especially if they were vomiting or had severe diarrhea. This time there had been no vomiting or diarrhea, so I was caught off guard.

Somehow we had been so focused on her not eating that we failed to note her lack of fluid intake. At 18 months most of her water came from pureed foods, and babies who aren't eating can become dehydrated rather quickly. The moral of this story is— carefully monitor your baby's fluid intake and retention, especially if he isn't feeling well.

Recovery Diet

After a digestive disorder take special care not to give a child food that will irritate his stomach. Warm foods and drinks are gentler on the stomach than cold ones. If vomiting has been severe, it may take extra time to adjust to a normal diet.

Begin by trying sips of the following liquids:

- Warm tea or water
- Pear juice
- Chicken or beef broth (see below)
- Thin rice cereal

As he begins to recover, these foods are appropriately mild:

- Bananas
- Chicken
- Applesauce
- White rice
- Lean beef
- Toast without butter
- Baked potatoes without butter
- Peppermint drops are soothing and good for children who are old enough not to aspirate them.

Avoid all milk products and fatty foods.

Space meals 5-1/2 hours apart.

Chicken Broth

Chicken broth is a wonderful food for ailing stomachs. It is gentle on the tummy and contains a lot of protein from gelatin boiled off the bones.

1. Place whole chicken in large pot; add enough lightly salted water to cover it; boil for at least 1-1/2 hours.
2. Pour off broth and cool to room temperature..
3. Refrigerate until fat congeals on surface.
4. Skim off fat and serve warm.

Antibiotics and Intestinal Disorders

If a child is running a fever with an intestinal problem, he may need antibiotics after the vomiting has stopped (see Chapter Seven).

For persistent diarrhea but no fever or vomiting, first try an enema. Make sure the enema is followed by a gentle diet (See pages 78-79) If the enema and soft diet do not cure the diarrhea, the next step is to determine whether your child's intestinal tract is reacting to a particular food. Ask the question, "Has he eaten anything unusual or new recently?" Maybe he is allergic to something.

If you cannot pinpoint any particular food that could be causing the diarrhea, it is probably wise to try an antibiotic. It's possible to have an intestinal infection, even without fever. Erythromycin (see pages 104, 109-110) is an effective antibiotic for intestinal infections. If the diarrhea is not at all affected by the antibiotic, the child may need testing at a hospital.

Note: For information on preventing infectious intestinal disorders, see How to Stop Passing the "Bugs" Around, pages 105-106.

℘ 5 ℭ
Fever

Esther's temperature was 105.5°. I stared at the thermometer in disbelief. What if it kept rising? What if she didn't recover? Panic rose in my chest as I looked at my little daughter lying listlessly on the couch. Her complexion was frightfully pale against her dark curls. The usual cheery smile had disappeared, and her normally sparkling eyes were dull and glassy. Oh, how I wanted my bouncy Esther back again! After five anxious days her temperature dropped, and as Dr. Denmark predicted, she broke out in a rash typical of German measles.

Fever can be frightening. High temperatures are also a blessing, however. They are the body's alarm system, alerting us to sickness. There is hardly a child who never experiences a fever. Every mother needs to know how to diagnose and treat it.

Diagnosing a Fever

When a child is uncharacteristically fussy and warm to the touch, take his temperature. If you are using a digital thermometer, consult the accompanying directions in the box.

For glass thermometers, use the following procedure:

Procedure

Rectal (infants and toddlers)

1. Shake the mercury down.
2. Lay baby over your lap and gently insert the thermometer one inch into his rectum.
3. Pinch buttocks gently around the thermometer to keep it in place and hold for one or two minutes before reading.

Underarm (young children)

1. Shake the mercury down.
2. Place the bulb of the thermometer in the child's armpit.
3. Bring the arm down over the end of the thermometer and hold securely for two or three minutes. Try to keep the armpit airtight.

Oral

For older children who will not bite the thermometer or break it.

1. Shake the mercury down.
2. Place the bulb of the thermometer under the tongue and instruct the child to keep it there with his mouth closed for one to two minutes.

One degree above the following readings indicates a fever: under arm (97°), oral (98.6°), rectal (99.6°).

Fever is caused by infection. Scientists aren't certain what it does but have observed that different germs cause fever with varying characteristics. With a strep infection, the temperature typically runs low in the morning and may even be subnormal before noon. Then it usually begins to rise, peaks at 6:00 p.m., and goes down around 2:00 a.m.

Fevers accompanying flu or German measles tend to remain fairly consistent throughout the day. A fever brought on by an abscess usually drops when the abscess is opened.

Treatment

If your child registers an abnormal temperature, first check him for meningitis (pages 47-48). Meningitis is always an emergency. If the fever's cause is not evident, periodically check for its symptoms. If any symptoms of meningitis are present, go immediately to the hospital. When meningitis is ruled out, look for the following:

- A cold (pages 89-90)
- Swollen glands in neck under jaws (pages 96-97)
- A throat redder than the color of his gums (page 96-99)
- Pulling at ears (pages 94-96)
- Stomachache (pages 51-52)
- Diarrhea (see Chapter Four)
- Vomiting (see Chapter Four)

If an intestinal disturbance is evident, an enema is probably in order (see Chapter Four). If symptoms are mild, inconclusive, and/or indicate an upper respiratory problem, the following are recommended:

1. A hot bath. Run the shower first so the room will be warm and steamy. Dry him off and dress him in pajamas from another room so his clothing will be dry.
2. Aspirin (dosage indicated on next page).
3. Bundle the child up. When he starts to perspire, usually around the back of the neck, begin taking layers off. Change wet clothing.
4. Continue to observe the child for a rising temperature and other symptoms.

Aspirin Dosage

(Low dose 81mg chewable tablets originally called "baby" or "children's" aspirin)

1–3 months: Mix one crushed baby aspirin and five teaspoons water; give one teaspoon.

3–5 months: Mix one crushed baby aspirin and four teaspoons water; give one teaspoon.

5–7 months: Mix one crushed baby aspirin and three teaspoons water; give one teaspoon.

7–12 months: Mix one crushed baby aspirin and two teaspoons water; give one teaspoon.

12 months: One whole baby aspirin. If he won't swallow a tablet, crush it and mix it with water or honey.

2 yrs to under 3: 1-1/2 baby aspirin tablets

3 yrs to under 4: Two baby aspirin tablets

4 yrs to under 6: Three baby aspirin tablets

6 yrs to under 9: Four baby aspirin tablets

9 yrs to under 11: Four to five baby aspirin tablets

11 yrs to under 12: Four to six baby aspirin tablets

12 yrs to adult: Five to eight baby aspirin tablets

Adult: use adult aspirin, and consult bottle for dosage

Note: Aspirin should be administered every four hours as needed. It is a safe medication that has been used effectively for over a hundred years. Dr. Denmark did not believe that aspirin causes Reye's syndrome (for further discussion see pages 72-73, 102-103).

Note: Four baby aspirin equals one 325 mg. adult aspirin.

With a high fever a child has chills. Many infants and toddlers will sit in their mothers' laps and want to be cuddled for warmth. Applying cool cloths to the child's forehead or cool baths is not recommended. Cold baths may cause a seizure.

Boy, I'm going to meet "they" someday and really get educated. A woman called the other day with a baby who had a fever. "Give the baby a little aspirin," I said.

"They say you shouldn't give a baby aspirin," the mother said.

I said, "Then why'd you bother me? Do what 'they' say. If 'they' know what to do, why bother Dr. Denmark and waste her time?"

Fever and Enemas

A fever may inhibit digestion and thereby cause vomiting and diarrhea. Enemas will help. They can actually help reduce any high fever by replenishing vital body fluids. Sometimes aspirin may be added to the enema if the child cannot keep it down orally (see Chapter Four).

Diagnosing the Severity of an Illness

Every child's reaction to infection is individual. Some typically run higher temperatures than others. One may have a low fever and be very sick, though another's temperature may spike with the least illness. Some have a tendency to complain intensely with the least discomfort, while others hardly complain at all, even when they are very sick. Our Leila can spike 105 degrees and still be coherent, while Steven has been delirious at 101 degrees.

You need to evaluate the child's general behavior to determine the severity of the ailment. Observe his appetite, playfulness, and coordination in addition to his temperature, and compare his behavior to what it normally is.

Your instincts are often accurate. If you're worried and not sure what the problem is, consult a physician. Any high or prolonged fever may indicate a need for antibiotics (see Antibiotics, Chapter Seven).

Lots of kids get "busitis." They wake up in the morning desperately ill. As soon as the school bus leaves, there's an amazing recovery!

Recovery

It's easy to assume a child is well when his temperature is down in the morning. However, temperatures due to staph and strep infections characteristically drop in the morning even before true recovery. Just because he appears well, don't send him back to school or take him to church. Going into public too soon may prolong illness and infect other children. The child's white blood cell count may be low, rendering him more susceptible to picking up something else. He should have at least two fever-free evenings before resuming his normal routine.

ᥱ 6 ℆
Infectious Diseases

Steven announced dramatically, "I'm sick and need to see Dr. Denmark." He trudged into the living room toting his plastic doctor's kit. I was clearing the lunch dishes. Out of the corner of my eye I saw him fluff a pillow on the couch, climb aboard, and pull a blanket up to his chin.

Methodically, he felt his forehead and stuck the toy thermometer in his mouth. When the kitchen was clean 20 minutes later, I brought a basket of laundry into the living room to fold. He was still lying on the couch with the toy thermometer protruding from his mouth.

"Are you still playing doctor?"

"I have a throat infection," came the muffled reply, teeth clenched around the thermometer.

"You poor baby," I crooned. I walked to the couch and laid a kiss on his forehead. It was warm. I felt his neck.

"Steven," I remarked in surprise, "You do have a sore throat." His brown eyes looked puzzled.

"I told you I was sick."

Our children are generally very healthy, but we aren't exempt from colds, sore throats, and the like, especially during winter months. Common illnesses can become serious if not treated properly. With Dr. Denmark's help I learned to diagnose and treat them.

Today young pediatricians tend to avoid treating their patients until an illness is severe. That's not my way. In my opinion, if a physician sees something wrong, he ought to take care of the problem before it becomes severe.

Aspirin is recommended throughout this chapter to combat fever and aches. Dr. Denmark did not believe that aspirin causes Reye's syndrome (See pages 72-73, 102-103). **Refer to Chapter 9 for information on recommended medications.**

Diagnosis of Common Illnesses

Carefully observe your child's behavior and apparent physical condition. Look for specific symptoms to indicate the problem.

- Fever
- A throat redder than his gums
- Swollen neck glands
- Congestion
- Runny nose
- Coughing
- Pulling at ears
- Stomachache
- Abnormal stools with an unusually strong odor
- Diarrhea
- Vomiting
- Rashes
- Loss of appetite
- Headache
- Inconsolable crying
- Burning sensation when urinating
- Lethargy and weakness
- Unusual crankiness

Normally, symptoms will indicate one particular illness, but occasionally a child may be fighting more than one at a time. For example, he may have flu and chicken pox at the same time. He could be battling an infected ear and food poisoning concurrently. Both illnesses must be treated at the same time. Dr. Denmark preferred broad-spectrum antibiotics, and these are effective in treating a variety of illnesses simultaneously. Also, her schedule for administering antibiotics should be carefully followed (see Chapter Seven).

Symptoms may be inconclusive. If there is no emergency (see Chapter Two), you may have to wait a few hours until more definitive indications surface.

Years ago when I first started practicing medicine, if a doctor didn't know what was wrong he would say the patient was bilious. Biliousness wore out. Now doctors just say it's a virus. Now everything is a virus.

Colds

A child with a cold needs care to prevent secondary infections of sinus, ear, and throat. Keep him warm, give him plenty of fluids, feed him well, and help him rest. Aspirin* will make him feel better and reduce inflammation. If he's very congested, clean out his nose so he can breathe better.

Procedure

1. Twist a piece of sterile cotton onto the end of a Q-Tip so that it hangs approximately an inch off the end of the stick.
2. Dip the end of the cotton into Argyrol* or saline solution (1 tsp. salt per quart of water) and squeeze off excess.
3. Twist the end of the cotton into the child's nostril (only the cotton should enter the nostril) and pull it out. Repeat for other side. Use the procedure once daily for **no longer than three days.**

Sitting in a steamy bathroom can also relieve congestion. Close the door, turn the shower on hot, and stay with the child until he is breathing more easily. Dry him off and dress him in clothes from another room so that the garments will be dry.

Don't use a vaporizer. Vaporizers or humidifiers increase the moisture in the house and encourage the growth of mold, a common allergen. If necessary, use a dehumidifier.

Note: We have also used Chlor-Trimeton or Benadryl syrup* to relieve congestion from colds. It can be used in conjunction with aspirin.

I'll tell you how those cold-air vaporizers got started. Years ago mothers noticed that if their babies had the croup, rocking them on the porch helped. No, it wasn't the cold air that enabled them to breathe better—it was the clean air. Everyone inside was smoking.

Once I was notified that a patient in the hospital with croup was desperately ill. When I arrived, I found they had put the child in a tent, breathing ice cold mist.

"Take that baby out of there," I said to the nurse. "Bring me a rocking chair and a blanket. Let mama roll him in it up good and tight and rock him for a while." Within a few minutes the child was much better. There's no excuse for a cold air vaporizer. Nobody in his right mind would go to a cold, wet climate to get well.

Never use a suction device in the nose. If your child's nose is running clear, it probably indicates an allergy (see Chapter Eight). If the discharge is not clear, he has a sinus infection. A fever with the cold may indicate a secondary infection. If he has a fever in the morning, give him a hot bath and aspirin* and observe him. Should his condition worsen by afternoon, you may want to see a physician and use antibiotics.

With any excessive or persistent fever, notify a physician.

Coughing

Never use cough medicine. When the cough reflex is suppressed the lungs can fill with fluid, and pneumonia may develop. Coughing, sneezing, and runny noses are nature's way of cleaning out the system. An expectorant or decongestant should not be used either.

Coughs often get worse at night or early in the morning when the child first wakes up, often due to postnasal drainage.

If a minor but persistent cough keeps him awake, try giving him something sweet. A little sugar, Karo syrup, or a peppermint drop might help. (Exercise discernment concerning the age of your child before giving him a peppermint. A young child risks inhaling it.) The sugar makes saliva flow and dilutes the mucus which may be causing the cough.

Aspirin* is also effective in treating a minor cough caused by postnasal drainage. It helps dry up the drainage and reduces swelling in the nasal passages. Chlor-Trimeton or Benadryl syrup* may also be used to treat this type of cough.

With excessive, deep coughing, the child should see a physician (see Whooping Cough, pages 103-104, Pneumonia pages 93-94).

Even if a baby's coughing at night bothers you, never give him cough syrup. No, no! If it bothers you so much, maybe you parents should consider taking something to get to sleep!

Wheezing

Wheezing when breathing **in** indicates croup. Take the child into a steamy bathroom. Give him a hot bath and aspirin*. An antibiotic may be needed with fever (see Antibiotics, Chapter Seven).

Wheezing when breathing **out** indicates asthma. It is produced by allergens and the cause(s) should always be investigated (see Allergies, Chapter Eight). Give the child aspirin, warm or hot water to drink, and an antibiotic if there is fever. Do not use a vaporizer.

Flu

Symptoms are headache, fever, and chills. Fever can prevent proper digestion of food, so the child may also suffer intestinal distress. Be sure he stays warm and well hydrated. Encourage him to rest and keep him at home, isolated from other germs. Aspirin* may be used for fever, and enemas are useful in combating vomiting and diarrhea. Flu takes the following course:

Day One: The child is miserable with fever, chills, headache, and possibly digestive disorders.

Day Two: Feels better.

Day Three: Feels considerably better and will often want to resume a normal schedule. Unfortunately, it is on the third day that the white blood cell count drops drastically. At this time resistance to secondary infections is almost nil. Before antibiotics were discovered, death was not uncommon from secondary infections contracted in the aftermath of flu. He should be pampered for a week after symptoms have subsided to allow time for his resistance to build again.

Antibiotics are often needed to prevent secondary infections. Ampicillin* is recommended.

There is no effective immunization against flu simply because one can catch it repeatedly. Immunizations only work against diseases like whooping cough that give lifetime immunity.

I learned the truth of Dr. Denmark's caution concerning secondary infections the hard way. Joseph came down with the flu one summer while he was part of his brothers' lawn business. He felt pretty rotten and lay in bed for a few days. After the rest, Joseph was so much better that I encouraged him to get back to work mowing lawns. His brothers needed his help—or so I thought.

It wasn't long before his fever was up again and this time it developed into a deep cough. An x-ray verified that he had pneumonia. This time it took much longer for him to recover, even with antibiotics. His cough lingered for weeks. Don't underestimate the effects of flu on your immune system.

Pneumonia

As a rule, children don't get pneumonia unless they have taken cough syrup or have accidentally aspirated something into their lungs, causing infection to develop. A child can also catch pneumonia as a secondary infection from the flu (see previous page).

Symptoms are fever, coughing, and rales in the chest that are detectable through a stethoscope. But often you can hear them by pressing your ear against the child's back, under the shoulder blades, and instructing him to breathe deeply. If he has pneumonia you'll usually hear a "sticky" sound as he inhales. The sound is similar to that of a lock of hair being rubbed between the fingers. Pneumonia is serious. If you suspect your child has it, consult a physician. Penicillin* should be administered around the clock for at least seven days. Never give cough syrup.

There's no such thing as "walking pneumonia." Well, I take that back. If he has pneumonia and walks to the bathroom, you could say he has "walking pneumonia." If someone walks in my office there's "walking pneumonia." You see, it would be the same pneumonia if he was in bed. I guess there could be "automobile pneumonia." It all depends on how you're getting around!

Sinus Infection

Infection develops when allergies or colds cause the walls of the nasal cavities to stick together. The sinus cavities then become stopped up and abscesses form. Some children's temperatures may climb as high as 106°. If a screaming child has yellow mucus draining from his nose, he likely has a sinus infection. The sinuses, however, may become so stopped up that there is no drainage at all. Clean the nose with Argyrol* or saline solution to reduce swelling (See page 89). If the child develops a fever, get a prescription for penicillin or ampicillin*.

To avoid such infections, try to determine the causes of your child's allergies and keep him away from them. Common allergens are pollen, smoke, and dust from carpets.

Infected Ears

If a child complains of earache, particularly after swimming, press the V-shaped protrusion on the outer part of the ear (above the earlobe next to his cheek). If pressure increases the pain, he's likely to have swimmer's ear, a fungal infection that requires a prescription from a physician. In contrast, pain from an abscessed ear will not typically increase with such pressure. It can actually give some temporary relief.

Dr. Denmark recommended aspirin* and Auralgan* for pain. To administer Auralgan, turn the child on his side and release several drops, squish them into the ear by pressing gently with your fingers. The effect lasts about four hours. Auralgan does not combat infection but is merely analgesic.

Use ear drops only when there is pain. Sudden relief of pain or blood may indicate a ruptured eardrum, which normally heals within three days without causing deafness. Should the eardrum rupture, put nothing in the ear.

With very young infants, extreme caution should be exercised in using Auralgan. Ruptured ear drums are more difficult to detect in smaller ears.

Note: Do not confuse Auralgan* with Argyrol*. Auralgan is fine to use in the ears but highly dangerous to the nose or eyes.

If the child runs a fever with an earache or the earache is especially severe, he may need ampicillin or penicillin*.

Frequently a younger child will cry with an earache until he sits in your lap and presses his ear against your chest. The pressure relieves the pain and quiets the child. If he's put back into the crib, he may begin crying as the pain again intensifies.

Tubes

Allowing tubes to be inserted into a child's ear can actually introduce infection and will permanently damage the eardrum. Tubes are not curative; they merely relieve some of the pressure caused by abscesses resulting from stopped-up eustachian tubes.

It is far wiser to cure the abscesses with antibiotics and determine what caused the eustachian tubes to stop up in the first place —commonly colds, allergies, and adenoids. **Consumption of milk products** and placing babies on carpets often contribute to congestion and ear infections (see Allergies, Chapter 8; See pages 241-244).

If a child is old enough to follow instructions to "sniff" in very hard, it sometimes alleviates the earache by clearing the eustachian tubes. Dr. Denmark's system of administering antibiotics every three hours around the clock is a wonderful weapon against chronic ear infections. (see Antibiotics, Chapter 7)

If you were a drummer and someone bored a hole in the top of your most expensive drum, could you ever make it perfect again? I doubt it. You would have to purchase a new top for it.

Puncture an eardrum and there will always be scar. Some patients come to my office with pus running out of their ears and down their necks. They were unaware of having infected ears because there was no pressure from the abscess against the eardrums. The pus had made its way around the tubes.

Plastic surgeons try to rebuild eardrums that have been destroyed. Tubes are a money-making thing, but they have never helped any child under the sun.

Strep Throat

If any "healthy" throat is cultured it will show evidence of strep. When the body is run down, tired, hungry, or constipated, it can't resist the infection. Every bad throat is strep except in the case of diphtheria. When a child has a fever, one of the most common causes is an infected throat. Temperature begins to climb around 6:00 p.m. and goes down around 2:00 a.m. To diagnose, check with a flashlight for signs of redness and swelling. If the throat is darker in color than the gums, that probably means infection. To see more clearly, you may have to depress the tongue with a spoon and instruct the child to say "ahhh."

Another method is checking for swollen glands. Hold the back of the neck and head with one hand and instruct the child to lift his chin slightly. With the other hand, feel under the jaw for swollen glands. They feel like large marbles.

Treatment

Paint the throat with Mercurochrome or Merthiolate* once a day for **three days** to kill germs and reduce pain.

Procedure

1. Twist a piece of sterile cotton around a Q-Tip and dip it in Mercurochrome* squeezing off excess until it's almost dry.
2. Depress the tongue with a spoon; have the child say ahh," and dab the inflamed area. You may need a helper with a flashlight.

Gargling

Gargling twice a day with Listerine* or salt water can help. Saline solution: one teaspoon of salt to one quart of water. Any higher concentration can blister the throat. The child may need antibiotics if he is running a fever. They may also be in order if the sore throat is particularly painful and persistent, even in the absence of fever. Penicillin* works best for throat infections.

Most of our serious diseases are a result of three problems: (1) bad throats, (2) bad teeth, and (3) poor diet. Throat infections can affect other organs if they remain untreated and should be taken seriously.

Tonsils

Tonsils are organs in the back of the throat that are absolutely necessary to the infant during his time of nursing. They come together with the uvula as the baby is sucking. When he takes a mouthful of milk, the tonsils move back, the adenoids keep milk from going into his nose, and he swallows it. After the nursing period, tonsils normally atrophy.

There are large crypts in the tonsils which make them balloon if strep or staph goes down into them. Abscesses that medicine can't reach form in the bottom of the crypt. When the medication series is completed, germs migrate back to the tissue, and the child becomes ill again. The problem is similar to that of an abscessed tooth. It's impossible to get medicine into it.

After scarlet fever the tonsils may become infected with hemolytic strep that causes an enormous amount of pus, evident when they are pressed. The child will never be totally well until the tonsils are removed.

A tonsillectomy is also necessary if the child has a mouth-breathing problem or has had scarlet fever and later begins running a fever regularly in the afternoon, indicating rheumatic fever. (Normally adenoids should be removed with the tonsils.)

A little patient had her tonsils removed. The physician inadvertently left behind a tiny piece of tonsil that had a tiny white abscess on it. She developed a big knot in her neck and began to have swelling. We found albumin in her urine, indicating nephritis.

"If you remove the remaining piece of tonsil, the child will recover," I told her doctor. He didn't think it was large enough to be significant. The child became so ill that as a last resort, he finally did it. She began to recover and was completely well within a month. A tooth infection is like that tonsil. It's not much bigger than a pinhead, but it sure can wreak havoc in the body.

In the past, children with Down's syndrome drooled until we learned to remove their adenoids. When the adenoids were gone, they could breath through their noses and they stopped drooling.

Christina and Leila came down with scarlet fever when they were five and seven. Their temperatures skyrocketed to over 105°. With penicillin administered round-the-clock (See page 108) the fevers went away, but they were left with swollen tonsils and recurring sore throats. Dr. Denmark recommended tonsillectomies.

The hospital staff was wonderful and allowed us to stay with them until they were sedated. Surgery went smoothly and recovery wasn't so bad, especially with all the cold treats, get-well gifts and extra attention. I fondly remember them lying side-by-side on the top bunk delightedly licking popsicles. Their little sister, Susanna, confessed quietly to me, "I wish I could have my tonsils out, too."

Scarlet Fever

Scarlet fever is a hemolytic strep infection. Its symptoms are usually a bad throat, high fever, and a rash. If you rub your hand over the child's body, the rash feels like chill bumps. The skin on the abdomen may appear pink but not show a definite rash. The tip of the tongue and the roof of the mouth may be red. Penicillin* is generally prescribed.

Occasionally a child may have scarlet fever without a high temperature. If he exhibits other symptoms of the disease, see a physician immediately. Scarlet fever is a serious illness.

After recovery, periodically check the child's tonsils for signs of infection (See page 98).

German Measles

The symptoms of German measles are headache, high fever, and swollen lymph nodes on the occipital ridge behind the ears, as with chicken pox. Fever may run continuously for five days. On the fifth day a rash breaks out, usually starting behind the ears and moving to the chest. It then spreads over the entire body. The fever characteristically stops at that time. The rash may not disappear for three to four days, but once it appears the child is no longer contagious. Until the rash breaks out, you can't be certain what the child has, so antibiotics are prescribed early on. Ampicillin* is most often used when symptoms are not conclusive. Don't treat the rash, and it's all right to bathe the child.

Chicken Pox

Chicken pox begins as a red rash, round and flat, that develops into elevated bumps with clear blisters on top. There may also be swollen lymph nodes on the occipital ridge behind the ears. The blisters are terribly itchy for seventy-two hours and generally spread all over the body. The full breakout takes three days. The first day the blisters are clear; the second day they turn yellow; and the third day they become scabby and brown. They remain for sixteen days.

The incubation period is 16 days after exposure. A child is not contagious until he breaks out. He should then be isolated from other children. If you know your child has been exposed, isolate him on the 15th day after exposure and keep him isolated until you're sure he's not coming down with the illness. No one knows how long an individual with chicken pox remains contagious.

Fever does not accompany chicken pox unless there are excessive pox that inhibit perspiration, or an infection in the pox. Aspirin* can help with fever or pain. If the child runs a high fever, antibiotics may be in order.

Treatment

(**shingles** or **smallpox** can be treated the same way)

1. Keep the child from getting too hot; heat intensifies itching.
2. If the child perspires a lot, dab the pox gently with alcohol or witch hazel to prevent infection.
3. Keeping the child dry inhibits bacteria growth and helps prevent secondary infection and scarring. Don't allow the blisters to get wet for sixteen days. Never use anything abrasive to the skin such as oatmeal baths or other similar treatment.
4. Don't allow him to scratch; keep him covered and clip his fingernails very short.
5. Dabbing the blisters with Caladryl or calamine lotion* reduces itching. It may be applied repeatedly as needed.
6. Give Chlor-Trimeton or Benadryl* syrup every eight hours to relieve itching.
7. If pox get infected, apply Silvadene cream* twice a day directly to the individual lesion, but don't slather it on.
8. If necessity demands wiping pox on any part of the body, be sure to use sterile cotton moistened in sterile water. With girls, if there are pox in the vulva, wipe off the urine.
9. If the child's throat is affected, paint it with Mercurochrome or Merthiolate* (See page 97 for procedure).
10. Offer the child diversions—videos or crafts.

I saw a baby with chicken pox just the other day who had been treated with oatmeal baths. He had gotten impetigo and had blisters as big as silver dollars all over his body from infected pox. Keep them dry and they seldom get infected.

One year we battled six bad cases of chicken pox, five simultaneously. The children were terribly itchy and miserable for three days and nights. We dosed them with Chlor-Trimeton* around the clock and applied Caladryl* nonstop. One of us was holding the baby most of her waking hours to keep her from scratching.

It was hard to keep the baby's pox cool and dry in the diaper area. I put her in cloth diapers (pinned loosely with no plastic pants) and changed her as soon as I detected wetness. When she soiled herself I wiped her carefully with sterile water and sterile cotton and dried her with fresh cotton. She was congested and had a tendency to drool onto her chest. I kept a cotton bib on her most of the time, changing it and her T-shirt frequently. After meals I wiped around her mouth carefully with sterile water and sterile cotton, always drying with fresh cotton.

After the pox began to heal, I had to resist a mighty urge to ignore Dr. Denmark's advice and give them all a good scrubbing in the tub. I could hardly wait for them to be clean again!

Steven didn't share my sentiment and rather enjoyed his reprieve from soapsuds. At last, I happily ushered him into the bathroom and turned on the water.

"Wait, Mommy!" he cautioned, desperately searching for a pox on his stomach. "I'd better not have a bath yet. I'm sure there is still a pox somewhere!"

Do you know why people are afraid to give aspirin with chicken pox? It's because of that case a number of years ago which was so highly publicized. There was a child who had chicken pox and went on to develop diarrhea and vomiting. (Diarrhea and vomiting are not symptoms of chicken pox, of course. Something else was going on.) Anyway, the intestinal symptoms lasted for about four days, and the child's temperature skyrocketed to 106°.

On the way to the hospital, the child evidently was given one baby aspirin. By the time they took the child to the hospital, it was so dehydrated that it had Reye's syndrome. The Reye's syndrome was obviously due to prolonged vomiting and diarrhea, but they blamed it on the aspirin. There was something terribly wrong with the child if he had a 106° temperature with chicken pox. It may have been encephalitis or septicemia. However, aspirin is not what caused the Reye's syndrome (See pages 72-73).

Urinary Tract Infections

If a girl complains of a burning sensation when urinating, first check for redness in her vaginal area. Make sure she isn't bathing in bubble bath or using too much soap when she bathes. She may just need to rinse more thoroughly with clear water.

Children should not drink anything other than water. Fruit juice produces alkaline urine that can irritate sensitive vaginal tissue, makes children susceptible to urinary tract infections, and sometimes causes bed-wetting. Note that constant itching in the vaginal area may eventually lead to masturbation. If the condition continues after taking the above precautions, or she is running a fever with the same symptoms, she should see a physician and have a urinalysis done.

Macrodantin* (an antibacterial medication) is effective with urinary tract infections (cystitis).

Dosage for all ages: one teaspoon at each meal three times a day for seven days without stopping until the last day is complete.

Whooping Cough

Whooping cough is a serious, highly contagious disease of the respiratory system which can be prevented by timely vaccinations (see Immunizations, page 43-45, Ch 13). Children with whooping cough have severe, often frightening coughing attacks every four hours as their bodies try to expel thick globs of egg-white-like mucus. The child will choke, gasp for breath, and may even have convulsions brought on by a lack of oxygen to the brain. There is no fever unless a secondary infection develops.

Erythromycin* must be given for seven days.. It may be necessary for you to make the child gag and cough up mucus before medicine dosages so he will not cough the medicine up. Stimulate the cough by swabbing his throat with a wet cotton swab.

Never use cough syrup. It can actually cause pneumonia (see Coughing, page 91). Even if a child has recovered from whooping cough, he may continue to get bad coughs every time he has a cold for up to one year (see Chapter Thirteen and pages 256-259).

Cystic Fibrosis

If your child has chronic respiratory and digestive problems, it may be wise to check for cystic fibrosis. Cystic fibrosis is a hereditary disease in which the cells of mucous membranes in the body secret large amounts of mucus. Many organs may be damaged by this accumulation of mucus, primarily the respiratory and digestive systems.

You can determine whether your child has this disease in 24 hours with a simple test. Cut a square of photo film and insert it inside the child's recently expelled feces. Wrap the specimen up tightly and put it aside for 24 hours. Then wash the film and look at it. If the film has become clear, then the child does not have cystic fibrosis because the feces contains the necessary enzymes to digest protein. If the film remains unchanged, then the child lacks those enzymes and likely has cystic fibrosis.

Dr. Denmark recommended that a child with cystic fibrosis be given regular doses of pancreatic granules and papaya juice. He should also be served a low protein diet and no milk products. A physician needs to be consulted immediately.

How to Stop Passing the "Bugs" Around

Occasionally one of our children will bring home a highly contagious "bug" and it's passed through the family. Battling such illnesses can be extremely trying for everyone. We really make an effort to avoid picking up and passing the bugs around!

Healthy children are less likely to catch something. Develop good health habits (see Chapter Eleven). Instruct your children in the practice of good hygiene. Washing hands frequently, covering the mouth when coughing, and not sharing cups are some of the obvious rules.

Avoid chills. Be weather-sensitive when you dress your children. Cotton undershirts in winter are good for girls as well as boys.

Separate sick children from healthy ones as much as possible (this is difficult). Certainly do not let them sleep close together.

Keep your kitchen surfaces and bathrooms disinfected and floors clean. When we moved to our present home we replaced carpets with wood parquet and linoleum. Since then we have had significantly less respiratory illness. It is much easier to keep wood and linoleum dust free and clean. I washed my nastiest laundry (diapers, wipe cloths, etc.) with a germicide and rinsed thoroughly to prevent allergic reactions to detergent or germicide. If the baby was sick we sometimes washed and disinfected his toys, too.

You cannot keep your children in a "bubble," but you can avoid taking little ones into public when there is a lot of illness around. Don't drop your little ones off at day-care or "mother's morning out." Hire an occasional baby sitter instead. Try not to use nurseries. Don't take sick children to church, and sweetly encourage your friends not to, either.

One fall our whole family attended a great conference. Unfortunately, an intestinal bug came home with us which passed through the family not once, but several times. I was desperate. Dr. Denmark instructed me to wipe all the handles and door knobs in the house with alcohol. We placed a hand sanitizer (62% alcohol) on the back of each commode. Everyone was told to use it after a bowel movement even before touching the toilet handle. I used the sanitizer immediately after cleaning vomit or changing diapers. We finally stopped passing the bug around.

*For information on recommended medications and substances refer to the following pages:

Medication	Page	Medication	Page
Argyrol	125	Kenelog cream	126
Ampicillin	125, Ch 7	Kwell	123
Aspirin	119-120	Listerine	123
Auralgan	125-126	Macrodantin	126
Benadryl	121	Mercurochrome	123
Bleach	127	Milk of magnesia	124
Caladryl lotion	121	Nystatin powder	126
Calamine lotion	121	Pedialyte	124
Clor-Trimeton	121	Penicillin	125, Ch 7
Dramamine	122	Silvadene cream	126
Erythromycin	125, Ch 7	Vermox	127

❧ 7 ☙
Antibiotics

"Steve, I took John and Susanna to Dr. Denmark today. They have bad throats, and she has put them on penicillin. Will you help me tonight? If you dose them at twelve o'clock, I'll do it at three. Don't forget to reset the alarm clock for me. You know what Dr. Denmark says about missing a dose!"

I've talked to scores of moms who are skeptical of antibiotics. They have related story after story of children taking them for weeks, even months. Often their pediatricians have tried several different kinds, progressing from cheap to very expensive varieties. Still their children do not respond. I hear of maintenance dosages, tubes in the ears, yeast infections.

It's a mystery to me why pediatricians have departed from the original system of administering the antibiotics that Dr. Denmark used. Instead of the typical four doses per day for ten days, we follow Dr. Denmark's preferred regimen. As a result, our use of antibiotics is short-lived and highly effective. In over 30 years our 11 children have never needed tubes in the ears and have almost never had relapses. I seldom have had to repeat a round of antibiotics. This mom is convinced that the original way is the best.

Effective Use of Antibiotics

Antibiotics kill bacterial cells by several methods, one of which is to keep them from multiplying. To be most effective, the medication has to be kept in the bloodstream by dosages given at **regular intervals around the clock**. Missing one by fifteen minutes can greatly decrease the medication's effectiveness. If they are always given on time you can expect to see a difference in your child's condition in 36 to 48 hours. If the child is recovering from flu, it may take a little longer. The regimen must continue for at least 72 hours, but it is seldom necessary beyond that. Occasionally a repeat of the whole treatment cycle is indicated.

The following are lists of the medications and dosages Dr. Denmark used most frequently:

Penicillin

Penicillin is most effective against throat and sinus infections; pneumonia; bladder, kidney, and breast infections; scarlet fever; and sometimes impetigo.

Dosages* (based on mg concentrations)
0–4 months: 125 mg (1/2 teaspoon)
4 months–1 year: 125 mg (1 teaspoon)
1 year–adult: 250 mg (1 teaspoon or one tablet)
Adult: two 250 mg tablets for the first eight dosages (every three hours) and switch to one 250 mg tablet for the remaining 48 hours

*Every 3 hours for 72 hours (around the clock).

Note: With pneumonia, dosages continue for at least seven days.

Note: If the child is allergic to penicillin, ampicillin may often be substituted.

Ampicillin and Amoxicillin

Ampicillin is most effective in the treatment of ear infections, flu, and meningitis and can also be used as an alternative to penicillin. Children usually prefer the taste of ampicillin, so it is easier to administer. In case of a fever without other conclusive symptoms (not clear what kind of infection is present), it's best to use ampicillin. The dosages for ampicillin are identical to those of penicillin.

Erythromycin

Erythromycin is most effective in the treatment of digestive problems like diarrhea and salmonella poisoning and can be used for whooping cough.

Dosages* (based on mg concentrations)
0–4 months: 200 mg (1/8 tsp) or 125mg (1/4 tsp)
4 months–1 year: 200 mg (1/4 tsp) or 125 mg (1/2 tsp)
1 year–adult: 200 mg (1/2 tsp) or 125mg (1 tsp)

*Every 3 hours for 72 hours (around the clock).

Note: With whooping cough, dosages continue for seven days.

If the child vomits the medication within 20 minutes, repeat the dose. If there is no more vomiting, continue schedule. Should it continue, stop the medication and try to determine the cause for the vomiting. The child may need an enema, highly effective in such cases. He may be allergic to the medication. In any case the vomiting must be stopped before an antibiotic can be effective. Erythromycin can give children a stomachache. If it's severe, cut the dosage in half.

Allergy to Antibiotics

An allergic reaction to medication is indicated by immediate and repeated vomiting, diarrhea, or rash. A rise in temperature is not symptomatic of an allergy. If you suspect an allergic reaction, discontinue it immediately and contact a physician.

Administering the Antibiotics

Doing it Dr. Denmark's way is admittedly more difficult than the four-daily-doses routine. It is critical that the medication be given precisely on schedule, so it takes discipline on the part of the parents—remembering to set the alarm, getting up in the middle of the night, dealing firmly with a sleepy, resistant child. Inconvenience, however, is a small price to pay for the benefits received.

I usually dose at hour multiples of three: 3:00- 6:00- 9:00, etc. I find it easier to remember this schedule when I'm sleepy.

Tips for Giving Medicine to Young Children

Ask your pharmacist for the best-tasting brand of a particular medicine. I use an oversized dropper that has a rubber ball on the end and is specifically designed for infants. These are available in most drug stores. They minimize spilling and enable you to coax medicine down the child more slowly. For older children I recommend a medicine spoon made in the shape of a tube ending in a "duck bill." If your infant (0–4 months) is taking erythromycin, you may need to purchase a 1/8 tsp. measuring spoon.

Since liquid antibiotics must be kept in the refrigerator, it's colder than a young child is used to. Fill the tube with a dose, put one finger on the end to keep the medicine from spilling, and run hot water over it. That takes the chill off and makes it more palatable.

Some children resist no matter how much they're coaxed or how good-tasting the medicine is. Keep in mind that they are simply too young to understand its importance. There are times a parent must be absolutely firm.

When we first began using antibiotics, patients went to the hospital every three hours for an injection. The results were miraculous. Later we discovered that taking oral doses every three hours was as effective. As time went on physicians decided adhering to a strict three-hour schedule was too much trouble. Besides, parents didn't like waking up at night and, well, it messed up a doctor's practice. It's not financially advantageous if patients recover quickly! But there is simply no way for an antibiotic to be effective unless it is kept in the bloodstream.

ဆ 8 လ
Allergies

"Dr. Denmark,…it's our twelve-year-old…she's broken out all over with a rash like small welts except on her face. New clothes? Well, she did wear a new outfit yesterday, and no, it's never been washed. You're saying she may be allergic to the dye? She does have very sensitive skin."

Identification

The day a person is conceived, lifetime allergies are established. One doesn't develop allergies or grow out of them. They can't be cured, but allergens can be avoided.

Allergy may manifest itself in a variety of ways, including respiratory problems, hay fever, vomiting, diarrhea, migraine headaches, eczema, rashes, clear runny noses, stomachaches, and asthma. It can produce different symptoms at different times. One day a child may have a headache and at another time break out in a rash in reaction to the same allergen. (Typically, fever is evidence of infection, not an allergy.)

Treatment

The first step is to discover the cause (or causes) and keep the child away from it. Use a process of elimination and closely observe him.

Common sources are mold, pollen, smoke, dust, milk products, citrus fruits, and chocolate. If your child is allergic to dairy products, remember that milk is not the only food to avoid. Dairy includes cheese, yogurt, sour cream, cottage cheese, and even whey. Most margarines actually contain a little dairy, so make sure you read the ingredients. It's difficult to find recipes that do not include dairy products, but a mother should persist for the sake of her child's health. Eliminate possible food allergens for at least two weeks before you rule out a particular food.

Carpets and rugs contain many allergens, so wood floors are much preferable to wall-to-wall carpeting. If your family has a problem with allergies, you might consider replacing carpets with linoleum, tile, or hardwood. Never put an infant down on a carpet even with a blanket beneath him. It can cause congestion and lead to ear infections. Don't use a humidifier because it produces mold. Keep the house as dry and dust free as possible. Use a **dehumidifier** if necessary. Prohibit smoking indoors.

Avoid the use of lotions, powders, creams, and perfumes and **rinse soap thoroughly** from skin and clothes. Use a pure soap such as Ivory, or try a variety until you find one that works well for your child's skin. For a child with sensitive skin, wash new clothes before he wears them (See page 58).

Mothers long ago didn't know the word allergy, but they might say, "Every time he goes to the hen house he gets the wheezies." Another might observe, "Every time he goes to Grandma's and sleeps in the feather bed, he gets the wheezies." Observation is a key ingredient to determining allergies.

Most congestion is a result of an allergic reaction to tobacco smoke, pollen, and mold. During rainy weather a lot of children get stopped up noses. If parents use a vaporizer, the moisture level in the house is increased, producing more mold. The only place steam should be used is in the bathroom with the door closed.

In years gone by we sent children to the desert or to the seashore to cure respiratory problems. The ocean air was fresh, and beach houses had open windows, spotless linoleum floors, and little dust or mold. It was easier for allergy-prone people to breathe in those environments. When reading the Old Testament we find that the Israelites burned down houses that had mold growing in them. They knew it would make them sick.

"Mommy, I feel like there are spiders crawling around in my covers." (John speaking)

"Did you roll around in the grass outside today?"

"No."

"Did you get a shower this evening?"

"Yes."

"Hmm, let me look at your sheets...I don't see anything..."

At first it seemed like a ploy to delay bedtime, but this kind of conversation occurred frequently, along with the complaint of itchy undershirts, necklines, and socks. We tried switching soaps and shampoo with no success. Finally, after I changed to a new brand of laundry detergent the "spiders" went away. We'll probably never know exactly what it was, but there was something in the old detergent John was allergic to.

Allergies and Infants

Careful observation of a baby on breast milk can identify allergies early on. If he exhibits allergic symptoms, experiment with eliminating various foods from your diet.

Introducing baby foods too early doesn't cause allergies, but don't do so before 12 weeks in any case. An infant isn't able to digest foods properly before then. At 12 weeks the child typically begins to drool, indicating his saliva now contains ptyalin, an enzyme that enables the liver to change starch into sugar. Digestion of food begins in the mouth and is not possible until drooling begins. Now begin giving him one new food at a time with careful attention to possible allergic reactions. If a child is allergic to a particular food, he is allergic to very small amounts of it, not just large amounts (See page 29).

An allergy is like stealing. If you take a penny, you might as well have taken a million dollars—it's still sin. A mother says, "Oh, I didn't give him enough to hurt him." She gave him a drop and his body reacted. You can't play around with an allergy. If it's wrong, it's wrong.

Desensitizing Shots

Test series may be helpful in determining allergies, but shots are not effective. If a child receives a skin test series, the mother can try exposing him to some of the substances his skin has shown a sensitivity to. Some of the substances may cause a visible allergic reaction; others pose no problem at all. But the best solution is to discover the allergen and stay away from it.

It was useful to discover through skin testing that our Christina is allergic to cats—at least some of us were glad to find this out. The cat lovers in our family were distressed and would rather we had stayed ignorant. "Sorry, no kitties allowed inside."

My husband had severe allergies, so we routinely avoided taking any room on the first floor of a hotel. We knew from experience that the rugs there would be musty. The higher the room, the less mold and dust. We also discovered he was allergic to raw apples. Every time we visited one of his sisters, he came home terribly ill. Though he could eat cooked apples, we finally determined the culprit was the raw ones in her wonderful Waldorf salad.

Antihistamines and Decongestants

Chlor-Trimeton syrup (see page 121) is a good antihistamine. Do not, however, use a decongestant. The body tries to expel foreign matter in the same way eyes tear to expel sand or dust. A decongestant hinders that process.

Emergency

Some allergic reactions are life threatening. If your child begins to have respiratory problems or has welts covering his body after a bee or wasp sting, take him immediately to the emergency room. With any severe allergic reaction, don't hesitate to consult a physician.

❧ 9 ❧

Dr. Denmark's Medicine Cabinet

"Mommy, I hate to wake you up, but I can't sleep. My ear is killing me. Can you give me something to make it feel better?"

"Don't worry about waking me, Jessica. It must hurt pretty badly. I'll get Auralgan and aspirin from the medicine cabinet. If it's not much better by morning, we'll have Dr. Denmark take a look at it."

Illnesses and injuries are unpredictable, so every mother needs a locked medicine cabinet stocked with some basic supplies. The following is a list of medical supplies and medicines Dr. Denmark used. Some dosages are also given. For use of the medicinal items, refer to preceding chapters.

Nonprescriptive Items

Aspirin

—for colds, fever (see Chapter Five), headache, earache, menstrual pain, pain due to minor injury, or fever from vaccination. It does not cure infection, but it is a pain and fever reducer and is anti-inflammatory.

Dosage

(Low Dose 81 mg chewable tablets originally called "baby" or "children's" aspirin.)

1–3 months: dissolve one crushed baby aspirin in five
teaspoons of water; give one teaspoon.*

3–5 months: dissolve one crushed baby aspirin in four
teaspoons of water; give one teaspoon.*

5–7 months: dissolve one crushed baby aspirin in three
teaspoons of water; give one teaspoon.*

7–12 months: dissolve one crushed baby aspirin in two
teaspoons of water; give one teaspoon.*

12 months: One baby aspirin.* If your 12 month-old will not
swallow a tablet, crush it and mix it with water or honey.

2 years to under 3: 1-1/2 baby aspirin tablets

3 years to under 4: Two baby aspirin tablets

4 years to under 6: Three baby aspirin tablets

6 years to under 9: Four baby aspirin tablets

9 years to under 11: Four to five baby aspirin tablets

11 years to under 12: Four to six baby aspirin tablets

12 years to adult: Five to eight baby aspirin tablets

Adult: use adult aspirin and consult bottle for dosage

*Aspirin should be administered every four hours as needed. It is a safe medication that has been used effectively for over a hundred years. Dr. Denmark did not believe that aspirin causes Reye's syndrome (for further discussion see pages 72-73, 102-103).

Note: 4 baby aspirin equals one 325 mg. adult aspirin

Caladryl or Calamine Lotion

(calamine 8%, pramoxine HCI 1%)—for itching due to insect bites (See pages 63-64) or chicken pox (See pages 100-103).

Apply as needed to reduce itching.

Chlor-Trimeton

(chlorpheniramine maleate) or **Benadryl Syrup** (diphenhydramine HCI)—for bee stings (See page 63), poison ivy (See pages 58-59), discomfort from chicken pox (See pages 100-103), or minor coughs (See page 91); congestion (See pages 89-90); allergic rashes (pages 58-59)

Chlor-Trimeton **syrup** is not commonly available. We order a chlorpheniramine maleate syrup through our pharmacy. It is called Aller-chlor and is manufactured by Rugby. Contact a pharmacist to order, or use a Benadryl syrup. If your child cannot tolerate Benadryl and you cannot obtain the chlorpheniramine maleate syrup, try crushing part of a Chlor-Trimeton tablet and mixing it with water, corn syrup or food. One teaspoon of chlorpheniramine maleate syrup is equal to 1/2 of a 4 mg Chlor-Trimeton tablet.

Dosage*

0–6 months: 1/2 teaspoon syrup or 1/4 of a 4 mg tablet
  crushed
6 months–adult: 1 teaspoon syrup or 1/2 of a 4 mg tablet
  crushed

* Normally administered every 8 hours as needed.

Cotton Swabs

—for treating infected throats (See pages 96-97), thrush (See pages 21-22), and cleaning out noses (See page 89)

Six-inch cotton applicator sticks are much handier to use than the more common Q-Tips but are more difficult to find. Ask your pharmacist for them or call a pharmacy that specializes in hospital supplies.

Dramamine

(dimenhydrinate)—for treating motion sickness (See page 53)

Enema Bag

—for administering enemas (see Chapter Four & kit instructions)

Purchase a douche-enema bag kit. These sometimes double as a hot water bottle. The ones I have seen most recently in pharmacies are made by Cara or Goodhealth. Not all pharmacies carry them, but they can order one for you. These brands work all right, but tend to leak after multiple uses where the enema nozzle (or pipe) screws into the tubing.

I prefer the fountain-style enema kits. We ordered a 1.5 liter fountain-style enema kit online at www.enemakit.com. The enema nozzle connects securely onto the tubing and does not leak. I also find it easier to clean. After using the kit, clean and store according to instructions on the box. I usually clean the pipe with alcohol between uses.

If you cannot readily obtain an enema bag kit and are in a hurry, purchase a larger, pre-mixed (saline laxative) Fleet enema. Even the adult-sized nozzle is small enough for a baby. Dispose of the solution, rinse the bottle, and use it in place of an enema bag.

Since the Fleet bottles are usually too small to contain all the Denmark enema solution, you will probably have to refill it and administer the enema more than once. After the bottle begins to collapse, it can help to withdraw the nozzle and unscrew the top so that the bottle fills with air and resumes its shape. Screw the top back, reinsert the nozzle, and squeeze out remaining liquid. **Avoid squeezing air into the rectum.**

Note: Dr. Denmark did not recommend the prepared, saline laxative Fleet enema solution for digestive disorders except for severe constipation.

Gauze, Band-Aids, Adhesive Tape

—for dressing minor injuries

Kwell

(lindane)—for treatment of lice (See page 65)

Listerine Anticeptic Mouthwash

—for alleviating sore throats (gargle twice daily)

Mercurochrome or Merthiolate

—antiseptic for cleansing wounds and swabbing throats (See page 97)

Unfortunately both of these medications are no longer being marketed in the U.S. They may be obtained from foreign sources.

(For substitutions refer to pages 128-129, 132-133)

Milk of Magnesia

(Magnesium hydroxide, 1200mg in each 15ml TB)—for minor stomachaches (See pages 51-52), mild diarrhea or constipation (See pages 71-72), and cleansing the digestive tract (See page 58).

Also used to prepare the digestive tract for an enema (See page 73).

Dosage
0–6 months: 1/2 teaspoon
6 months–6 years: One teaspoon
6 years–adult: Two teaspoons

Pedialyte

—for restoring electrolyte balance and preventing dehydration

It can be used effectively at any age (See page 77).

Rubbing Alcohol

—for cleansing wounds and disinfecting door knobs, handles, and commode seats. It is good to use when there's a lot of illness in the house (See pages 105-106) or when traveling.

Special Medicine Spoons

(See pages 110-111)

Sterile Cotton

—for wiping diaper area in newborns, cleansing wounds, cleaning out noses, opening tear ducts, and swabbing throats

Thermometer (mercury or digital)

—for taking body temperature (See pages 81-83)

Although mercury thermometers are more accurate than digital, they are much more difficult to find. Mercury thermometers are no longer sold in the U.S.; some foreign pharmacies may sell them via the Internet. For instructions on using a mercury thermometer, refer to page 82. After use, wipe it with alcohol, then wash with soap and cool (not hot) water.

For use and care of digital thermometers, consult the accompanying directions.

Vaseline (petroleum jelly)

—for applying to nozzle of enema tube and helping chapped skin (See page 62).

Witch Hazel

—for cleansing, and itching due to insect bites (See pages 63-64), chicken pox (See pages 100-101), or cleansing sunburn (See page 61).

Prescriptive Items

Antibiotics

(penicillin, ampicillin, erythromycin)—for infections diseases (see Chapter 7)

Argyrol

—Silver Protein—for eye infections (See page 66) and cleaning out noses (See page 89).

Argyrol is presently unavailable on the general market. However, some compounding pharmacies will formulate Argyrol.

(For substitute refer to pages 128-129, 132)

Auralgan

(Antipyrine, Benzocaine, and Anhydrous Glycerin)—analgesic for earache (See pages 94-95)

Auralgan should never be confused with Argyrol. It is obtained by prescription in the United States. In some other countries, it is a non-prescriptive item. Research this via the internet.

(For substitute refer to page 131)

Kenalog Cream

(triamcinolone)—for treatment of eczema (See page 57) 0.1% Kenalog cream would have to be obtained at a compounding pharmacy.

Macrodantin

(nitrofurantoin)—for treatment of urinary tract infections (See page 103)

Nystatin topical powder

(Mycostatin powder), 100,000 USP units/gram—for diaper rash (three times a day—see pages 27-28), eczema with a fungal infection (See page 57), athlete's foot (See page 60), or ringworm (See page 60). Nystatin powder is only available by prescription in the U.S. In some other countries it is a non-prescriptive item and low cost. Research this via the internet.

(For substitute refer to pages 129-130, 133)

Nystatin oral suspension

(Mycostatin suspension)—for thrush (See pages 8, 21-22). (For substitute refer to page 130)

Silvadene Cream

(1% Silver sulfadiazine cream)—for promoting healing whenever there is a break in the skin. Ask your physician for a prescription. **(For substitute refer to pages 129, 132)**

Vermox

(mebendazole)

—for treatment of pinworms (See pages 69-70)

Available Kitchen Items

Baking Soda

—for enemas

Salt

—for sore throats, tea enemas, cleaning out noses

Karo Syrup

(light corn syrup)—for tea enema

Black Tea

—for tea enema

Bleach

(regular strength: 5.25% sodium hydrochlorile, 94.75% water) —for bee stings, ant bites, poison ivy, athlete's foot, jellyfish stings, burns.

Note: Whenever bleach is used for treating the above, it must be rinsed off **thoroughly** to avoid blistering the skin.

I've used these medicines since they were made and those that work I continue to use. New medications are constantly being developed, and they're wonderful. But as long as my methods and medications are effective, why change?

Substitution Lists

(for hard-to-obtain medications)

It has been brought to our attention that some of the medications Dr. Denmark recommended are difficult to obtain, especially Argyrol, Merthiolate, and Mercurochrome which have been removed from the US general market. In an effort to make this publication more user-friendly, we have included lists of substitutions. We cannot claim that Dr. Denmark would have recommended the following lists. However, I have consulted with a friend and physician, Dr. Rhett Bergeron. Dr. Bergeron greatly respects Dr. Denmark's philosophy and incorporates many of her recommendations into his own practice. He is a traditionally trained medical doctor who also uses nutritional and natural medicines. At the writing of this edition, all of Dr. Bergeron's substitutions can be obtained at a health food store or via online sources.

Substitutions Recommended by Dr. Bergeron

For Argyrol, Mercurochrome, Merthiolate

Argyrol, Mercurochrome, and Merthiolate are all antibacterial medications. **Colloidal silver** serves the same purpose, is highly effective, and is non-toxic. Colloidal silver may be used to treat eye infections, swab throats, clean out noses, and cleanse wounds.

Dr. Bergeron notes some differences in the use of colloidal silver for infections and congestion. Because it is non-toxic, it may be used more frequently and for longer periods of time than Argyrol, Mercurochrome, or Merthiolate.

He suggests using it as eye drops one to three times a day for up to five days, depending on the severity of the illness (as opposed to the more limited use of Argyrol).

For treating sore throats, swab the throat or gargle with colloidal silver one to four times daily until redness and pain subsides. Gargling with silver is probably more effective, but swabbing can be used for children who are too young to gargle.

Use colloidal silver in the nose two to three times daily for up to ten days. Refer to page 89 for the procedure Dr. Denmark used or spray it in the nose with a nasal spray applicator.

Recommended brands for colloidal silver are Sovereign Silver and Argentyn 23. Dr. Bergeron emphasizes that homemade silver products should be used with great caution, the primary concern being silver toxicity.

For Silvadene Cream

Silvadene cream is also an antibacterial ointment. Dr. Denmark prescribed Silvadene for the treatment of any break in the skin. As an over-the-counter substitute for Silvadene, Dr. Bergeron recommends **applying colloidal silver, followed by Calendula cream mixed with lavendar oil**. For every one-half teaspoon of Calendula cream, mix in approximately one drop of lavendar oil. Apply the silver and the cream mixture with the same frequency as is recommended for Silvadene.

For Nystatin or Mycostatin Powder

Mycostatin powder is an antifungal agent. As a substitute for Mycostatin, one can use **Calendula cream mixed with tea tree oil, garlic oil, or oregano oil.** All three oils are antifungal. For every one-half teaspoon of Calendula, mix in one to two drops of oil. Sometimes a combination of two different oils can be mixed with the Calendula.

For example: 1/2 tsp Calendula

One to two drops of tea tree oil

One to two drops of garlic oil

Use with the same frequency as is recommended for Mycostatin.

Note: oregano oil is highly effective but has a very strong flavor, so it's best **not** to use it orally.

Where a combination of Silvadene and Mycostatin is needed, such as severe diaper rash, colloidal silver can be first applied, followed by a Calendula cream/antifungal mixture.

For Nystatin or Mycostatin Suspension

Nystatin Suspension is also an antifungal medication. Dr. Denmark recommended it for thrush. As a substitute, use **both colloidal silver and garlic oil.** First, dip a cotton swab in the colloidal silver and swab baby's mouth with it. Afterward, use another cotton swab and swab his mouth with garlic oil. Continue swabbing with both ointments after each feeding until thrush goes away.

Probiotic supplementation should always be considered in yeast infections such as thrush.

For Kenalog Cream

Kenalog cream was used by Dr. Denmark for short-term treatment of eczema. Kenalog is a steroid. **A mixture of lavender and rosemary oil mixed with Traumeel cream** is a good substitute for Kenalog.

Use:

1 tsp. of Traumeel
1 to 2 drops of lavender oil
1 to 2 drops of rosemary oil

Start by using one drop of each kind of oil and increase to 2 drops as needed, depending on the severity of the eczema and how it responds to the ointment. Use with the same frequency as is prescribed for Kenalog, alternating with colloidal silver when the eczema is infected. (See page 57)

Dr. Bergeron emphasizes the importance of determining the cause of the eczema. Often, it is a reaction to a food allergy. Dairy products, corn, wheat, eggs, and sugar are common culprits.

Note: Traumeel cream is also good for treating bruises, sprains, and muscular soreness.

For Auralgan

Dr. Denmark recommended Auralgan for ear aches. Auralgan is an analgesic and simply relieves pain. Use **Traumeel Ear Drops** instead. **Arnica, Beladona, or garlic oil drops** may also be used. Traumeel, Arnica and Beladona are analgesic whereas garlic has an antibacterial effect. A combination of drops can be used. For any of these remedies, **use one to three drops every one to four hours until pain subsides. Then, use one to two times daily for a few more days.**

For those families who do not utilize "natural medicines," we also consulted with my uncle, Dr. Jefferson Flowers.

Dr. Jefferson Flowers is board-certified in both family and emergency medicine. He has practiced for fifty-four years.

Substitutions Recommended by Dr. Flowers

For Argyrol

Dr. Denmark used Argyrol for eye infections and cleaning out noses. Dr. Flowers utilizes erythromycin drops for eye infections (a prescription item) and saline solution for congestion. Mix one teaspoon salt to a quart of water, bring to a boil, and cool completely. Use a few drops in each nostril as needed.

For Mercurochrome, Merthiolate, and Silvadene

Dr. Denmark recommended Mercurochrome and Merthiolate for cleansing wounds and swabbing throats. Dr. Flowers suggests first washing wounds with Ivory soap and warm water. If the wound is minor, instead of using Silvadene, simply apply one of three over-the-counter salves: Neomycin, Neo-polycin, or Bacitracin. These should be applied **two to three times daily** until healing is complete.

If the wound is more serious, follow the Ivory soap cleansing with Hibiclens (Chlorhexidine Gluconate 4%) Apply two to three times the first day after injury. Then continue with the salves.

These salves are good for most wounds, but Dr. Flowers claims there is really **no medication equal to Silvadene for burn treatment.** If a burn is more than light red, use Silvadene two to three times a day until healed. Keep the burn clean, but it's best not to cover it with a dressing unless there are blisters. Never attempt to break the blisters as they protect the skin from infection.

Instead of swabbing sore throats with mercurochrome or merthiolate, dissolve two teaspoons of salt in one quart of water.

Gargle with the solution two to three times daily. If soreness does not improve within a few days, antibiotics may be needed.

Dr. Flowers also highly recommends Mycolog cream (nystatin and triamcinolone—a prescription item) for diaper rash, eczema with a fungal infection, athlete's foot, ring worm, fever blisters, and cracked nipples when nursing. He calls it a "shotgun medicine" as it contains a blast of five different medications. Mycolog should be applied three times daily. For cracked nipples apply, wait fifteen minutes, and rinse with warm water before nursing.

Dr. Flowers treats poison ivy by having his patients wash the affected area three times daily with Ivory soap and warm water until the rash disappears. This cleansing removes the ivy oil and prevents rashes from spreading.

ಠ 10 ಠ
A Mother's Presence

The following was written many years ago when most of our children were very small. Friends warned me that time would go swiftly, and it has. Even with eleven children, babyhood seemed to fly by and now our home is filled with lively young adults.

I live amidst a happy beehive of activity, laughter, discussion, music, and sometimes arguments and tears. The dynamics and demands are different now. I am still busy, but I do have a lot of help with logistics. Our house stays cleaner, and occasionally I even take naps in the afternoon.

It has been exciting watching our children grow, mature, and develop talents. We have celebrated a myriad of birthdays, achievements, successes, marriages, and the birth of grandchildren. There has also been pain—something a mother cannot escape in a sinful world. Eve mourned her murdered son.[1] Even Mary's heart was pierced by a sword of agony.[2] We cannot escape all heartache, disappointment, fatigue, and grief that attends motherhood. Yet, for those who commit their mothering to Christ and follow His Word, there is a secure hope. Regardless of sin and mistakes, in the end, all shall be most well.

Dr. Denmark once said to me, "Mrs. Bowman, you really are a blessed woman!" She was right. Rearing eleven children hasn't been easy. Each of my *"olive plants"*[3] represents a challenge, but each also adds a richness to our family circle. For parents who know Christ, each child is a reward,[4] a blessing. When I meditate on the past, enjoy the present, and look to the future, I can honestly and joyfully echo what I wrote years ago:

I love being a mother. I love the oh-so-soft touch of a newborn's head against my cheek, nursing baby in my great-grandma's rocker, tickling little tummies fresh from the bath, the laughter of my little ones playing (and hopefully not quarreling) in the backyard. I love taking the kids for a walk on a beautiful afternoon—me pushing the stroller and excited children zooming around on roller blades. One of my favorite pastimes is sitting under our oak trees watching the little ones swing and show me what they can do on monkey bars.

It's great to see happy anticipation on faces when I cook something special for Friday evening. It's fun to braid the little girls' beautiful hair, help my kindergartner master his alphabet (he is so enthusiastic!), and eavesdrop on cute conversations among the children.

What could replace the precious voices when they are praying, reciting verses, or singing about Jesus? I would never trade the experiences of reading stories on the den couch, children running to greet me when I return from an errand, and all the kisses and homemade cards I receive on my birthday.

Yet we know that motherhood is not all peaches and cream. Who enjoys wiping up vomit off the floor, having to paddle so-and-so for the umpteenth time for the same offense, the anxiety when her fever shoots up to 105°. Nobody enjoys discovering someone very soiled who should have gone to the potty thirty minutes ago, slipping on legos while making a mad dash to the phone, or feeling very stretched when four voices are asking questions at the same time.

We live in a fallen world. We are sinners and our precious children are also. But somehow, God in His wisdom and mercy, brings all these experiences together to teach us, bind us together as families, and help us learn what it means to live for His glory. Through the curse of pain and struggles, He changes us, blesses, and brings joy in our sacred callings as mothers.

"Do you work, Mrs. Bowman?" When I'm asked that question, I'm tempted to be flippant.

"Work? Why, yes, as a matter of fact. I was up till four this morning with a sick baby and grabbed two hours sleep before my workday started again. No, I don't usually watch soap operas and eat bonbons. Challenging? Oh yes. I must stretch my capabilities to the limit. In my job, there are many hats to wear. I am counselor, doctor, teacher, nutritionist, housekeeper, drill sergeant, secretary, and watchdog all rolled into one.

Committed to staying at home? Yes, because I'm convinced my children need me. Despite all my faults and inconsistencies, I provide something no one else can, something they desperately need—a mother's presence.

A mother cat would never leave her kittens to someone else's care. Mother birds don't push their babies out of the nest until they are old enough to fly, yet an increasing number of mothers regularly drop their children off at day care facilities.

Daniel Wattenberg, a writer for Insight magazine, summarizes results of recent research on infant care. "Evidence is mounting that as the two-earner family has become the norm, parents may have compromised the early development of children. Infant day care is being linked to emotional and behavioral problems in children."[5] Jay Belsky, professor of human development at Penn State University and former proponent of infant day-care writes: "Children who initiated care in the first year...seemed at risk not only for insecurity but for heightened aggression, non compliance, and possibly social withdrawal in the preschool and early school years."[6]

According to Karl Zinsmuster, an adjunct scholar at the American Enterprise Institute: "The loving care of a biological parent, the mother nine times out of ten, is still the best care; accept no substitutions. The child, at least for that first couple of years, has to see a parent most of his waking hours...Apparently, infants cannot cope with regular extended separations in those first couple of years....There's just no evidence that you can raise children as a hobby on the side and have them come out right."[7]

Dr. Brenda Hunter, psychologist and specialist in infant attachment applauds stay-at-home moms. "These mothers are at home because they know that they, and not a child-care provider, can best nurture their children and give them a sense of home. They know children thrive in their mother's presence and suffer from her prolonged, daily absences....Babies need their mothers. They need them during their earliest years more than they need baby sitters, toys, or the material comforts a second income will buy."[8]

Infants are not the only ones at risk for lack of mothering. In Can Motherhood Survive?, Connie Marshner observes:

"Children in America are starving—for love, for attention, for their parents to notice them—not in a casual way, by giving them more toys. These children learn early that talk is cheap. 'I love you, dear,' from your mom doesn't mean much if you have to hang out at a neighbor's house to find someone who has time to listen to what's worrying you."[9]

Christine Dubois left an exciting job in a corporate office to care for her baby. "After two years away from the office, I still feel the lure of the fax machines and business suits," she reflected. "But I can honestly say I'd rather talk to Lucus than meet with VIP's, rather read 'Humpty Dumpty' than study top-secret memos, rather eat peanut butter and jelly than dine well during power lunches.

"My son is a different person than he was two years ago. And so am I. I've witnessed the everyday miracle of human development, been part of the wonder of discovering Lucus. I've fed and dressed, worried and laughed, comforted and cared. But most important of all, I was there."[10]

Moms, are you listening? Are you there to nourish with your presence and to enjoy the privilege of guiding and watching your children grow? If not, you may be missing the greatest moments of your life. Don't be duped by modern cultural pressures. Don't sell your birthright for a mess of pottage.[11] Make no mistake: Children can be frustrating and require a lot of work, but no occupation is without its moments of tedium. There is no greater privilege or more important occupation than being a mother at home.

Dads, are you listening? "Children spell love T-I-M-E."[12] Are you willing to embrace this high calling of your wife as being more important than having a second income?

Dr. Denmark believed it's absolutely critical to a child's health and well-being that mothers invest their time and energies at home, particularly when children are young. She, too, was highly disturbed over the increasing numbers of children who spend most of their waking hours in day care. Her counsel is encouraging, inspiring— and convicting. **(What follows is Dr. Denmark's counsel in her own words.)**

Responsibility

"Women have made and trained every man on earth except Adam. As women think and conduct their lives, so goes the country. Today women are brainwashed into believing there's some job in the workforce greater than being a wife and mother at home.

"'I'm not the type to be tied down with a baby and a home. I wouldn't be able to take it,' a woman once told me. Well, why did she get married and have one in the first place? I would never kill a baby under any circumstances [abortion]. If I were to put the baby on the counter and hand the mother a knife and say, 'Take its head off...' no woman would do it—not a one. She wants a law passed so somebody else can kill that baby for her, and then she's not to blame. We're looking for excuses in life all the time. If people don't want children, there are ways to keep from having them—like remaining single and living a chaste life.

"The issue is not capability—a woman is capable of doing most anything. But if she brings a baby into the world, she should take responsibility for it."

Education

"Someone brought me a book entitled, Why Would a Woman As Smart As You Be at Home? The theory is that if you have a wonderful education, you should go do something worthwhile with it and let lesser people rear your children. It won't work; it has never worked. A cow never neglects her calf. It would be enlightening for people to study how animals take care of their young until they are grown enough to take care of themselves.

"There's never been a woman too educated to take care of her baby. My mother cared for me, and I didn't have a bit better sense than to take care of my daughter. Mary had an excellent education and could have been a successful businesswoman, but she too stayed home and reared a couple of fine sons.

"America today is a wrecked nation. Eighty-five percent of our children go to day care and learn to fight their way through life. There, a child tries to build something and the other children snatch at it and tear it down. He in turn begins snatching and fighting. There is no peace for him. He's not able to have a quiet time at home. He'll not learn to do things by himself or learn self-discipline. He can't develop confidence in anyone because his mother has deserted him. Rejected youngsters will one day ruin our country.

"We must find women willing to stay at home and teach their little children how to read and write, how to stay in their rooms and build something. Children in day care learn to be robots; at home they can learn to be individuals."

Economics

"We've taken the baby out of the cradle and put the economy in it, setting him aside to make money. We're going to make careers and all kinds of things, but we're not making people. Somebody has to be willing to stay home and do that.

"You hear about so many women entering the work force. They think they've found freedom but don't seem to realize they aren't free at all. Working eight hours a day or getting fired makes them more like slaves. If they've earned a million dollars by the time they're sixty-five and never know the joy of rearing children, they haven't accomplished anything.

"I spoke with a woman not long ago whose baby had been in day care ever since he was six weeks old. It cost her four hundred dollars a month and another fifty dollars every week or ten days in doctor bills. The baby was constantly sick. [These figures are twenty-five years old. Day care and doctor's bills are much higher now.] She said she had no choice because she and her husband were buying a house. I asked her how long it would take. They had a thirty-year loan.

"That poor woman comes home every night tired out, to a tired husband and a sick baby. After thirty years, what will she have? She'll probably lose her husband, her house will be out of date, and she'll never have developed a good relationship with her child. She'll never have any of the wonderful pleasures of living. It's better to live in a lean-to and have some of the fun. We've somehow convinced working women they're having a good time. There's no good time to it at all."

Johnny's Day

"This is an example of the way thousands of little children are treated today by mothers who think homemaking is menial:

Mama and Papa, up at 6:00, must get Johnny up and bathed in a hurry, must get breakfast, and be at the office or other place of business by 8:30. Johnny gets up unhappy because he did not get enough sleep. Breakfast is rushed and forced on Johnny who will not eat fast or maybe not at all. Time is passing fast, and they must get to work; Papa and Mama get mad, talk loud, blame each other for not getting Johnny to eat. He is too upset to eat much or use the bathroom. At 7:30 the station wagon arrives, and he is rushed off without a good breakfast or elimination.

"Mama and Papa rush off to their separate jobs and work hard all day. Mama works for a handsome man who is dressed neatly and always seems to be in a good humor. She becomes dissatisfied as she compares her husband with the man she works for. Her boss has a good wife at home who looks after his children and his clothes and has time to see that he has good food served well. He feels that the money he makes is spent for a good cause and he is a happy man. The man she is married to could be happy if he had a wife who would make a home for him even though they would not be able to buy as many gadgets.

"She doesn't realize that her boss would act just like her dissatisfied husband if he were married to a working woman like herself. A good, homemaking wife is the best tonic to make a happy man.

"Papa rushes out into the office and he may become attracted to a beautiful girl working for him. She has attractive clothes, and is not so stressed. He may compare her to his wife who is trying to carry two full-time jobs. The single office girl is more relaxed, not too tired, has all the money she makes to buy clothes, take trips, and broaden her topics of conversation. She has time to read, keep up with the times, and is entertaining to be with.

"It might put Papa to thinking, 'If I were married to a girl like that, I would be happy.' (In fact, that girl would be just like his tired wife if she had him and his children and held down a full-time job away from home.)

"Little Johnny has been in nursery school all day among people with whom he would not dare be his normal self, for few children act up for anybody except their parents. The teacher will say, 'Mrs. Jones, Johnny is the best little boy I ever had.' But when Mama and Papa show up, he starts whining and showing his temper.

"Johnny's routine at the nursery runs like this: He gets there at 7:30-8:00; at 10:00 morning snack. (He did eat a few mouthfuls of food at breakfast). Lunch at 12:00, which he eats because he is afraid not to eat, and there is not anybody present he loves to whom he can voice his objection to food. So he eats it all. Naptime at 2:00, sleeps two hours, up at 4:00, has a glass of milk and some cookies. At 6:00, back in the station wagon and taken home.

"Mama, Papa, and Johnny arrive home, Papa tired and remembering how kind and nice the office girl had been to him and how good she looked when she left the office; Mama tired and conscience-stricken about her neglected child, but remembering how kind the boss talked and how patient he was. Johnny was fed four times during the day so has a stomach ache and is not hungry. He has slept all afternoon and is not sleepy.

"Now supper has to be fixed, clothes to wash and iron for tomorrow, baths to get, an apartment to clean as they did not have time to do these things before work. Now Mama says to Papa, 'I am just as tired as you are, so put that paper down and give Johnny his bath while I cook supper.' Johnny objects. He has not had a chance all day to show his willpower, for he could not do this to a person who is not a good audience. So the show starts. Johnny will not take off his clothes. Papa tries first to persuade, then to bribe, then to tease. When all that fails, he uses a loud voice and then the belt. That makes Mama mad so she comes in and finishes up the bath. The little fellow finds out he doesn't have to mind Papa when Mama is around.

"Supper is on the table, and it is a task to get Johnny in his chair. He had food just two hours ago, so doesn't want dinner. Papa serves his plate and Johnny pushes it back. Both Mama and Papa try all the tricks in the book to get him to eat but it does not work. Then they speak in cross terms to each other; Johnny is spanked and put down. Mama and Papa don't talk anymore until they have swallowed what food they have on their plates.

"They would like to get Johnny to bed, for housework would be much easier if he was out of the way. Meanwhile, he's crying, turning over chairs, turning up the TV, jumping off the best sofa, and slamming doors. He does all this to get attention and to show Papa that he can't do much about his conduct while Mama is around. (If the child is a girl, she shows Mama up, for Papa will be sorry for her.)

"Mama is conscience-stricken about poor Johnny because she knows she is neglecting him and she cannot stand to see him spanked by his father. She knows she deserves the punishment herself.

"Then they try to get Johnny to bed. He is not sleepy because he slept all afternoon. He is undressed by force and put to bed but he will not stay, calls for water time and again, then eventually just crawls out. They give up and let him stay up until they get the housework done, which is about 11:30. Then they all go to bed and sleep for six hours, provided Johnny will quit calling out, 'Mama don't leave me. Mama I don't want to go to sleep.'

"This is the life thousands of little children are living in our country today. How could we expect anything good out of children brought up like this?"

The Best?

"Many modern women are determined to provide everything for their children they didn't have when they were growing up. So they find outside employment.

"Is it best for children to have things or to be prepared to use things? Parents might be determined their kids are going to have good houses, cars, education. The best would be for them to teach those children a way of life; then they needn't worry about the rest. I've seen women in the slums who made their sheets out of rags, yet their children went to college.

"I made my way through college without asking my parents for help. What they gave me was a good start. If you give a child a brain you don't have to give him money; he can make it himself. It takes parental care and guidance for a child to develop to his full potential. If he hasn't the necessary mental and emotional maturity, all the money in the world won't enable him to make it in life.

"I don't believe anyone can be too poor to take care of her baby. One of my mothers bore a son out of wedlock. The father wanted nothing to do with her, so she was on her own. She cleaned houses to earn a living and took the baby with her in a basket while she worked. That woman kept her son with her until he was old enough to go to school. He turned out to be a fine young man.

"When I was a child, there were tenant farmers who worked for my father. The women worked with them in the fields, and they also took their babies along in baskets – no leaving them with strangers. My sister was a seamstress. She reared three fine children and never left them. She did her sewing at home."

Attitude

"A woman who would rather be doing something else can't be a good mother. Subconsciously, she'll hate her children because they prevent her from being a lawyer or a doctor or having a big time. I knew a great tennis player who put her baby in day care. If she felt tied down at home when she wanted to be on the court, do you think she would be good to her child? 'You children are depriving me of my game today.' That's the attitude many children are living under.

"The mental health of mother and child greatly depends on her attitude toward her vocation. Today, women have been brain-washed into thinking they've been abused since the beginning of time. They resent the fact that they've had to wash diapers, cook, and tend their babies. Nobody mentions how they got the money to buy the diapers and food. They forget about the poor man who plowed all day, wearing himself out in the cold and heat for the income to purchase essentials. We're telling women how abused they were in the past. It's simply not true. Theirs were the happiest homes in the world. Mama was doing what she loved to do, and her husband was making it possible for her to have what she needed."

Relationships

"The most important people in life are our little people, our husbands, and those who looked after us when we were young. Tragically, these are the three classes of people we have discarded. The old people are shut away in nursing homes. Men? We don't need them any more. We can handle our own business, and we're tired of them imposing on us, insulting us. Babies? When they turn six weeks old, we place them in someone else's care. Children are the sorriest, most neglected creatures we have on earth today.

"I see so many women who simply don't want to focus on their homes. They find something outside that they want to do. They've got to go do something 'worthwhile.' They are quite willing to teach other people's children or do volunteer work for a children's hospital, but they just don't want to be 'tied down' with their own children…the mother is out working for some other person, in an office, school, church, child guidance organization, child health organization, doing P.T.A or club work, or engaging in many other endeavors. She is giving her time and thoughts trying to make a better world for her child to live in, but is missing the only chance she will ever have to mold her child who is to live in the world she is trying to make. It is like a hen that will leave her little chicks out in the cold while she goes off to build a nest and finds, after the nest is built, her chicks have died from neglect.

"Did you read what Ann Landers wrote about me? She said, 'Dr. Denmark preaches that a woman should not pursue a career and look after her children, but Dr. Denmark is a professional woman herself.' Ann Landers didn't realize that I am preaching what I practiced. Sure, I'm a professional. I had plenty of help with housework, but my office was next to my home, and no one else looked after my daughter. I fed her and put her to bed; she played outside my window. I had breakfast with my husband and supervised things at home. I avoided the myriad activities other women doctors got involved in simply because my first obligation was to my family. I made a vow when I married Eustace that I would be a good wife to him. We had a glorious time together.

"I don't believe I would be able to handle my career the same way today and still care for a child. No, it would be impossible to be an attentive mother under present circumstances. Good domestic help is too scarce, and modern-day medical practice is structured differently.

"Incidentally, something has burned me up for years. My husband is the one who made it possible for me to practice medicine the way I have. I never had to worry about expenses or providing an income, so I could donate my time to the poor. If it hadn't been for Eustace, I wouldn't have been able to charge my regular patients so little. I've been awarded many honors, but he never received a bit of credit. He was responsible for any accomplishments I have attained. I couldn't have done it without him. Don't you think the Creator should be praised more than the created?"

Grandparents

"If a mother can't look after her children for some reason, then a working grandma should retire and do it for her. Had my daughter been unable to care for her sons, I would have given up medicine. It didn't mean anything to me in comparison to my grandsons. Unfortunately, grandparents no longer feel a responsibility to their grandchildren. They act as though they have paid their dues when it comes to child rearing.

"Grandparents are the Supreme Court for their grandchildren. They should model decent behavior, dress, eat, and speak well. Many aren't very good models. I see grandmothers coming to my office in tight, short skirts with cigarettes hanging out of their mouths. Nobody ever finishes paying his dues. People always have a responsibility toward one another, especially family."

Home

"All the women who have climbed to the top in society (in medicine, law, and business) and haven't had the experience of rearing their own children...well, when they turn 65 somebody will throw them a fancy retirement party; then they'll be left with nothing.

"I had a friend years ago who was a wonderful doctor, made a great income, and lived in a beautiful home. She never married. When she retired no one ever cared enough to visit her.

"'If you had your life to live over again, would you live it the same way?' I asked her shortly before she died.

"'No, I wouldn't,' she replied emphatically. 'I've never had any of the things that bring true happiness—a husband or a child. I've never really had a home.'"

Expert Advice and Parenting

"We have been duped into believing that no one knows anything but so-called experts—doctors, psychiatrists, news commentators. When I was a young doctor, I knew it all. Of course, I did because I had just finished medical school. I had all the answers, that is, until Mary was born.

"One of these highly educated, really important women called me the other morning. 'Dr. Denmark,' she said, 'I've been thinking about some of the advice you give on feeding children. You know the authorities think you are wrong. They say a baby should nurse on demand and children should eat six times a day.'

"'Just who on earth is the authority? That word is a funny one, isn't it?' I said to her.

"Mrs. Cow never asked Mrs. Pig how to take care of her baby. I believe a woman is as smart as a cow. Surely she can care for her baby as well as a cow looks after a calf.

"It's a queer thing—a cow never read a book, never watched a TV documentary, never read a parenting magazine or asked a doctor how to parent. I believe if we just use our heads, we can take care of our young instead of wrecking them as we do.

"When I was a young girl, there was a doctor who lived behind our property. Dr. Bowen was one of our dearest friends and later helped me through medical school. When one of the family was ill, he'd come over and ask my mother, 'Alice, what's wrong? What do you think we ought to do?' She'd tell him what she thought, and that's the way it went. Alice did the doctoring.

"A beautiful woman came to my office not too long ago with a baby who looked like the wrath of God. She was feeding it all day long and not having any fun. I questioned her about her background. Evidently, her own family had been terribly poor, but her mother had taken the time to prepare three decent meals a day. I looked at the woman and then back at her baby. That woman didn't need me; she needed her mother. If she'd listen to her, she could have a healthy baby just as her mother had. We don't need doctors any more; we need parents. Nowadays we have everything under the sun to keep children healthy—money, clean water, baby food, blenders, medicine—everything except parents.

"So many people today are like broken dishes. Individuals like the late Mother Theresa and James Dobson are trying to glue the pieces back together. Some of the plates will look whole and might even become usable. But wouldn't it be better to keep plates from being broken in the first place? If a mother stays at home and takes the time to care for her family, she's giving her child a chance to remain whole."

Notes

1. Genesis 4:25.
2. Luke 2:34-35.
3. Psalm 128:3.
4. Psalm 127:3.
5. "The Parent Trap," Insight (March 2, 1992), 6.
6. Jay Belsky, "Homeward Bound," Focus on the Family
     (January 1992), 7.
7. "The Parent Trap," 9.
8. "Homeward Bound," 6.
9. Connie Marshner, Can Motherhood Survive? (Brentwood,
     TN: Wolgemuth and Hyatt, 1990), 11.
10. "Romancing the Mom," Focus on the Family (February 1993).
11. Genesis 25:27-34.
12. Reverend Jerry White, Bold Ministries.

ॐ 11 ॐ
Nutrition and Health Habits

Reading books and articles on nutrition can be terribly frustrating for a mother. The nutrition experts change their recommendations every few years, or even months as new research is completed. Not only is the advice we receive through the media changeable, the prices at grocery stores are downright depressing. Does a family have to be wealthy to be healthy?

Dr. Denmark always emphasized the importance of good nutrition and a healthy life style, but conversing with her gave me the confidence that my children can be healthy if we stick to simple meals and common sense health habits. The excellent health Dr. Denmark enjoyed for over one hundred and ten years is convincing testimony to her understanding of what a body truly needs.

After many years in the practice of medicine, I have seen a great change in the problems that come to doctors. The tears that were shed for little children [at the early part of the twentieth century] were brought on principally by the ravages of disease-causing organisms that killed or left the children handicapped. Medical science has made great progress in conquering and reducing disease, but mothers still come with their tears. Now they are shed over the child who is a product of dissipation, born to parents who did not care enough to give the child the best possible prenatal start, and then the best possible environment that would make for as perfect a life as possible[1]... It seems that the human race has lost its knowledge and wisdom about how to care for the human body... A large portion of the doctor's time is spent trying to teach people what to eat or drink, when to eat or drink, and to patch up the bodies that have been damaged by dissipation and by improper feeding.[2]

Many people take better care of their cars than they do of their own bodies. They would never dream of using the wrong kind of fuel, yet consistently put the wrong kind of food in their mouths. Some families spend large amounts of money for all kinds of sweet drinks, milk, dry cereal, cookies, and many other things. That money could be spent for good meat, vegetables, fruit, and starches composed of whole grain breads and potatoes.

There are many products on the market today to make somebody rich and to destroy the person that is foolish enough to buy them. I hear parents in my office and in the clinic talking about how expensive it is to live and how little they have. As a rule, if they will go over the budget, they will find they are spending more to destroy their bodies than they are spending to build them up.[3]

Nourishment

Good nutrition is absolutely fundamental to health and happiness. A growing child particularly needs three balanced meals a day.

Protein

Each meal should contain high-quality protein. The best sources are lean meat, eggs, and black-eyed peas. All legumes have protein, but black-eyed peas have the most. Other legumes may be interspersed with meat and black-eyed peas. Lean red meat is healthful because of its high iron content. One egg a day won't harm anyone who is eating a balanced diet. Two eggs for breakfast are fine for children. For those who dislike eggs, it's all right to substitute other proteins. You can also disguise the taste of eggs in French toast (See page 164), or by boiling a beaten egg in oatmeal.

Don't be a slave to your child's desires, but exercise some creativity in encouraging him to enjoy healthful foods.

Incidentally, if anyone has difficulty getting moving in the morning, consider whether he is eating enough protein at supper.

During World War I, research was done on legumes and other meat substitutes. It was discovered that black-eyed peas had the most protein. We tried peanut butter—it's better than nothing, but it isn't as good as some of the other proteins. If you eat a good protein, you're not hungry till the next meal. However, if you eat a carbohydrate meal with no protein, you build a lot of insulin. On a breakfast of just a roll and orange juice, in two hours you have hypoglycemia. Then a teaspoon of sugar might keep you going beautifully for another two hours. It's killing you, but that's all right—the undertaker needs a job!

If you moved every time a child moved, I think you'd burn up a good bit of cholesterol. I see no harm in an egg; it's nothing but chicken. I've had an egg every morning for one hundred years. One a day won't hurt anybody.

No, I don't think there's anything wrong with eggs, but people do take things to extreme. I had a boy come to my office one day. He was 12 years old and weighed 225 pounds. I checked his blood pressure. It was 200/100. He was senile. I questioned him about his meals, and he said he ate a dozen eggs and a loaf of bread for breakfast. Everything that God made on earth, He made good. However, anything can be taken to extreme. Even water…you can drink enough water to commit suicide.

There's nothing wrong with red meat. It contains an enormous amount of the iron we need in our diet. At one point people wouldn't buy chicken because they didn't want the dark meat, so farmers started raising milk-fed chickens that were so anemic there wasn't enough red blood in the thigh to make it dark. The chickens had more white meat, but the thighs weren't as good food as they would have been had they eaten normally.

Starches

Every meal should contain a starch. Whole grains and potatoes are the best sources. Homemade whole grain breads and cereals are a great addition to any family's diet (See pages 172-173).

Whole grains are very important. Nowadays we take the vitamins out of food, put them into a bottle, and sell them.

Vegetables

At both lunch and supper, a child needs a serving of vegetables, especially green and leafy ones that contain iron. Spinach, collard greens, broccoli, cabbage, Brussels sprouts and romaine lettuce are some good choices. Alternate with yellow vegetables like carrots and squash. Though fresh produce may have a higher vitamin content, frozen or canned varieties are perfectly acceptable. Frozen vegetables are convenient and contain few additives or salt. Cooked vegetables are as good as raw ones and are actually easier to digest.

Hematocrits are done on children to show the number of red blood cells they have. It doesn't matter how many cells there are unless the cells contain enough heme to transport sufficient oxygen. Bringing a hundred empty train cars into a starving Atlanta would be purposeless; the cars have to be loaded with good food. It is the same with hematocrits. The amount of heme in the cells needs to be determined. People need the heme obtained from leafy green vegetables, lean meat, and whole grain bread.

Fruit

Fruit is not vital to nutrition. When a family is limited in its food budget, bananas and apples may be the best choices. Citrus tends to be overrated in its nutritional value. In years gone by, fruit was only eaten in season. Dr. Denmark's recommended diet for infants (See pages 28-37) contains a great deal of fruit simply because infants will eat vegetables and proteins more readily if they are mixed with fruit. Infants love food that is akin to breast milk. Like breast milk, it needs to be sweet and warm.

When I was a child we didn't have oranges in this part of the country. We each received an orange in our stocking at Christmas and that was all. So many times when people are grocery shopping they focus on oranges, grapes, and the like, but their money would be better spent for good vegetables, lean meat, and whole grain starches.

We've run this fruit business into the ground. Your great-grandma never had any fruit at all except in season. Fruit is all right, but there are other foods which are more necessary.

Sweets

Honey as a sweetener is far superior to sugar. Even sugar in limited amounts is not harmful to the average child. A sweet dessert once or twice a week won't hurt, but children should not expect to have them every day. Dessert on Friday night or for Sunday dinner makes the meal special and gives children something to look forward to.

Note: Do not give honey to a child under one year of age.

Everything's good until man makes it bad. There's nothing wrong with sugar unless it's eaten to excess. As a young person, I was a sugar addict. I began to develop arthritis at 35. My joints became sore, and I had pain in my hips. At 50 I eliminated sugar from my diet, and my hand is still as limber as any 16-year-old's. I can touch the floor without bending my knees.

I seldom buy candy, but when we have it, it disappears quickly. The older children occasionally purchase their own and stash it away in secret. When Joseph was a toddler, he was like a little bear with a nose for honey. No hidden stash was safe from his candy instincts. One afternoon I noticed the house was too quiet, so I went hunting for my little cub. After quietly opening the girls' bedroom door, I spotted Joseph at the far end of the room furtively devouring a box of leftover valentine chocolates.

When he realized he had been discovered and his time was limited, instead of repenting, the chubby hands began to move faster, desperately cramming the remaining chocolates into his mouth. By the time I reached him, both cheeks were bulging and thick brown, gooey drool streamed down his chest.

I took his sticky hand and led him toward the bathroom. He knew what was coming. "I'm sawee Mommy! I be a good boy."

Joseph, at 19, doesn't steal candy anymore, but I do occasionally find him nosing around the kitchen looking for something sweet. He's slender now, but I wonder what his girth will be 20 years from now.

Drinks

Don't drink anything but water, and drink when you're thirsty. So many are saying we need eight or more glasses of water a day. I don't think that's necessary. There is actually something called water intoxication. The blood can get so diluted that there are not enough electrolytes to make the heart beat (See page 22). We used to have a bucket on the back porch and people drank when they were thirsty. Individual needs can vary.

The family should not drink anything but water. Even fruit juices should be eliminated because of their concentrated fructose content. It's preferable to give a child fruit rather than juice. Fiber and protein in the pulp provide a much more balanced food. Juice stresses the kidneys and produces highly alkaline urine that can cause burning, itching, and even urinary-tract infections. Drinking water exclusively can sometimes cure a bed-wetting problem.

I wouldn't give a child anything to drink except water. I had a little boy in my office not long ago. He looked like the wrath of God. I tested his urine. I've never seen that much sugar in any human's urine. "Where in the world is he getting this sugar?" I asked his mother.

"We don't let sugar come into our house," she said. She was one of those health nuts.

"What does he drink?"

"Apple juice. I make it myself."

"What do you do with the pulp?"

"I throw it on the mulch pile."

I calculated that the child was getting eight ounces of pure sugar daily. I'm sure his eyesight was ruined.

"But it's natural sugar!" his mother said.

What sugar isn't natural sugar? The sugar mashed out of canes is natural. Everything on earth is natural! She was taking all the pectin, cellulose, and protein in that apple and throwing it away. The only thing the child was getting was the sugar and water.

People don't understand that children don't need juice. Why not buy the apple instead of just the juice? Why not buy the orange or the carrot and get the whole thing?

Dairy Products

Dairy products are much overrated in the American diet; they should never be a meal's main ingredient. Cheese isn't a good meat substitute; yogurt and cottage cheese are not much better. Milk consumption produces anemia. A little cheese sprinkled on top of a casserole, ice cream at a birthday party, or milk in a white sauce occasionally won't be harmful. But anyone past seven months shouldn't drink milk. Guard against regular consumption of dairy products in general. A good margarine is a better choice than butter. If a child is allergic to dairy products, even a small amount cooked with his food is detrimental to his health (see Index—Ear Infection).

My theory is that too much calcium inhibits absorption of iron. There has been a lot of research done on anemia. We know what causes it in calves—feeding them milk beyond the weaning point to make veal. It's not simply that the animal fills up on milk and neglects other food. We found that if a dog is given a pint of milk along with its regular diet, its hemoglobin drops ten points within a month. Some physicians claim that anemia is caused by bleeding from the colon. I don't agree. I believe it has something to do with absorption.

A three-inch square of cheese is equivalent to a glass of milk. A pizza contains a whole angle of cheese. It's one of the greatest assets to our medical profession. Pizzas produce more coronaries which in turn benefit cardiologists and surgeons. They make kids anemic and benefit pediatricians. Well, it takes the foolish to make the rich, rich.

When I was a youngster, we never saw milk on our table. Cows didn't produce much milk. Later, breeding produced cows which gave more milk and everyone started drinking lots of it. Then people began to develop pellagra.

We first began to buy loaf bread seventy years ago. At that time, "milk toast" became a fad. People would take a big slice of loaf bread, butter it, and toast it. They sprinkled sugar on it and poured milk over it. They might add a little vanilla or lemon to it. Well, people who ate a lot of it began to have diarrhea; they became anemic and started acting rather foolish. Some were actually sent to asylums. They had developed pellagra.

A doctor in Alabama began giving his pellagra patients cabbage pot liquor with wonderful success. We discovered that vitamin B, essential for good nutrition, was the missing ingredient in milk toast.

A mother brought her child in late one afternoon. She had had diarrhea for several weeks. The corners of her mouth were raw and bleeding. Her hemoglobin was 5. She should have died in her sleep. I didn't finish my examination but sent her directly to the hospital for a transfusion. This child had a severe case of pellagra. The mother informed me that she would eat nothing but cheese and white bread.

If I had a child like that, I would not say to her, "You can't have it." Instead I would say, "Sweetheart, we don't have any white bread or cheese in the house." Serve the right foods at meals, at the right time, and don't talk about it. I've never had any trouble feeding children.

Calcium

Calcium intake is much overemphasized. Most foods contain plenty of it.

A lot of widows develop osteoporosis in their old age, but it's not for lack of calcium. Without husbands to cook for, they snack and don't eat a balanced diet. Osteoporosis is caused by a lack of vitamin D necessary for the body's utilization of calcium. Vitamin D is obtained through sunshine, meats, vegetables, and codfish.

Fats

Avoid cooking with fat and cholesterol-laden oils, but a little vegetable oil for flavoring or even some bacon cooked with beans, soups, or greens isn't harmful. The key is moderation. When regular physical labor was a routine part of life, people could tolerate a higher fat content in their diets and remain healthy; it was burned off. Today we are too sedentary to consume much fat.

Mealtime

Meals should be spaced 5-1/2 hours apart, allowing time for the stomach to empty. If a child snacks throughout the day, that never happens. The stomach will not release undigested food other than sugar, so his body is unable to make use of what he eats, and he is constantly hungry. He also may be "pot bellied." Even nutritious snacks should not be permitted between meals.

Mealtimes should be happy, with your family sitting down together to thank God for the food and talking about the day. The dinner table is a wonderful place to draw closer, to learn and grow together, and to discuss spiritual truths and principles.

It's tragic that more and more families seldom eat together. There is no replacement for the fellowship, learning, and fun that happens around a table. When family members are too busy to share meals, they should reevaluate their priorities and time commitments.

At mealtime, it's best not to discuss the food (personal likes and dislikes). You needn't ask the children what they want or don't want; you can't be a short-order cook. The plates should be served with sensible portions of everything and placed in front of each child. If there is something all the children particularly dislike, use other foods of similar value; for example, broccoli instead of Brussels sprouts, raw carrots instead of cooked.

Don't ever say to your husband, "Forget giving Suzie her beans. She won't eat them." If you say that in front of her, she'll never eat them again. You can put ideas in children's heads. If they never know any better, they eat right. Once they discover refusing food produces chaos, they won't touch it.

I had a patient who wouldn't eat anything but corn bread. Well, his mother bought some baby food. She put pureed string beans and meat into corn muffins for her child. He ate them and had a good time.

A busy mom should focus on simplicity and good nutrition. There's nothing wrong with cooking more than enough for supper and having the rest for lunch the following day.

You needn't provide a gourmet meal every evening. It's fine to eat the same simple dishes often. They are less time consuming, more economical, and usually more healthful. Feasting should be reserved for special occasions.

Holidays were certainly times of feasting for our family when the children were young. My mother-in-law was of Lebanese heritage and a wonderful gourmet cook. "Sitti" (Arabic for grandma) and Granddaddy often had a fabulous Middle Eastern feast waiting for us when we arrived to celebrate. I encouraged the children to dress up, use extra-good table manners, help clear, and be sure to thank Sitti and Granddaddy before we left.

The event always began and ended with lots of kisses and hugs. I will never forget the little ones sitting around lovely tables set with china and candles, dressed in frilly dresses, smart little suits, and bow ties.

Little Jessica took after both grandmas in her flare for decorating and fashion. She also loved to make desserts. I complimented her once on a dessert she had prepared. Her smiling response was, "Yes, Mommy, the dessert is delicious. Sitti and I have good taste buds!"

Your great-grandma awakened and served breakfast at daylight. There was no refrigeration, and no one ate anything else until lunch at midday; likewise, supper. Those old people who were reared on three meals a day have tried dying at nursing homes. They built such good bodies they keep on living. Today we eat all day long, so kids are anemic and don't develop mentally as they should. Mother after mother tells me her family never eats in the morning. I can't imagine children getting up and not having breakfast with Mama and Papa before going off to school. Breakfast is the most important meal of the day.

Sample Menus

Breakfast (should include a protein and a starch)
- Boiled egg, oatmeal
- French toast with honey
- Fried egg, toast, banana*

It's best not to use milk in preparing French toast. Place a piece of whole wheat bread in a saucer and pour a beaten egg over it. Allow the bread to soak up all the egg. Fry it on both sides in a little margarine.

Lunch (should include a protein, starch and vegetable)
- Chicken sandwiches, green salad, apple*
- Black-eyed peas, brown rice, cabbage
- Lentil soup with vegetables, muffins

Supper (should include a protein, starch, and vegetable)
- Lean beef, potatoes, broccoli
- Baked beans, corn bread, yellow squash
- Beef stew, fruit salad*

* Fruits are the least important ingredient for a good daily diet.

In conversation with a young pediatrician at a medical meeting, I remarked that the most important thing a pediatrician should do is teach a mother how to feed and care for her children. I emphasized how much better it was to teach them how to keep their children well rather than simply hand them another prescription.

In response to my words the young man threw up his arms and said, "They don't pay us for that!"

You know it might be better to take a child to a vet. Vets insist on good nutrition for their patients. The vet is very cognizant of the fact that food means everything.

One-dish Meals

We eat a lot of one-dish meals. They are easy to prepare, simple to serve, and contain all the essential foods. Here are a few of our Dr. Denmark-approved favorites.

Beef Stew

Combine:

2 lbs. stew beef cut in 1 inch cubes
5 carrots sliced
1 large onion diced
3 stalks celery sliced
2-3 potatoes cubed
1 28-oz. can tomatoes (or fresh equivalent)
1 clove garlic crushed
2 bay leaves
salt and pepper to taste

Cook all day in a slow cooker.[4]

Lebanese String Beans

(can use peas or lima beans also)

Sauté two medium onions in olive oil.

Add:

1 28-oz. can tomatoes (or fresh equivalent)
2 14.5-oz. cans (or fresh equivalent) string beans
4 tsp. chicken bouillon powder
1 or 2 tsp. lemon pepper
1/4 tsp. pepper

Simmer until flavors are blended and vegetables are tender.

Add leftover pieces of beef, chicken, or 1 to 2 lbs. crumbled tofu.

Serve over rice.

Grandma Hart's Famous Noodle Soup

Simmer, covered for 1-1/2 hours:

1 large chicken
14 cups water
1 tbsp. salt
1/2 tsp. pepper
1/2 tsp. basil
1 bay leaf

Remove chicken and bay leaf; skim fat off broth.

Add to broth:

6 medium carrots, sliced
3 stalks of celery, sliced
2 onions, sliced

Simmer for 45 minutes.

While broth is simmering, cool chicken, debone and cut in bite-size pieces.

Add chicken and 3 cups of uncooked noodles to broth during the last ten minutes of cooking.

Sprinkle with 1/4 cup chopped parsley (optional).[5]

Six-layer Dish

Layer in order in a large greased casserole, seasoning each layer with salt and pepper:

4 medium potatoes sliced

2 cups frozen peas or other vegetable
2/3 cup uncooked rice
2 medium onions sliced
2 lbs. browned and drained ground beef
2 qts. canned tomatoes (or fresh equivalent)

Sprinkle with 2 tbsps. brown sugar.

Bake at 300° for 2-1/2 to 3 hours until rice and other vegetables are done.[6]

Chicken and Dumplings

Cover with water and boil for one hour:

1 whole chicken (4 to 5 lbs.)
1 chopped onion
1/8 tsp. cinnamon

Cool and debone chicken.

Skim fat off broth. (Broth should yield approximately 4 quarts.)

Add to broth:

1 package mixed frozen vegetables (or equivalent fresh)
3 cubed potatoes
chicken
salt and pepper to taste

Simmer for 25 minutes until potatoes are tender.

Make your own dumplings* or use canned refrigerator biscuits cut into fourths.

Drop dumplings into vegetable-chicken mixture. Cook 10 minutes uncovered and 10 minutes covered. Add them while vegetables are still cooking to save time.

*Dumplings:

3 tbsp. shortening or margarine
1-1/2 cups flour
2 tsp. baking powder
3/4 tsp. salt
3/4 cup milk

Cut shortening into flour, baking powder, and salt until mixture resembles fine crumbs. Stir in milk.

Beef and Rice Burritos

Cook 1 cup brown rice (yielding 2-1/2 cups cooked).

Brown together:

1-1/2 lbs. ground beef
1 chopped small onion
1 chopped green pepper
2 cloves garlic crushed

Drain and stir in:

1 tsp. salt
1-2 tbsp. chili powder
3 tsp. cumin
1 15-oz. can black beans (drained)
1 14-oz. can diced tomatoes or diced tomatoes with green chilies undrained (or fresh equivalent)

Cook mixture over medium heat for approximately 5 min.

Stir in hot cooked rice and spoon into tortillas. Wrap and eat.

Complete Meal Bean Dishes

We eat a lot of legumes for economy and nutrition. I often do them in a pressure cooker or a slow cooker all day. Black-eyed peas and lentils soften more quickly than other legumes. Here are some of our favorite bean recipes.

*Prep for dried beans:

Wash and sort beans, picking out the disfigured ones.

Put beans in a saucepan and cover with about two inches of fresh water.

Boil for 2 minutes.

Turn off heat, cover and let sit for one hour or soak overnight.

Drain liquid. Beans are ready to cook.

Note: Cook times for pressure cookers are indicated below. Follow manufacturer's instructions.

Cook times for slow cookers vary depending on the cooker. Set slow cooker temperature on high for most bean recipes.

Black Beans

Combine in pressure cooker (or slow cooker):

1 lb. dried black beans, prepped*
6 cups chicken broth
1 onion chopped
3 carrots sliced
1 bay leaf
1 tsp. oregano
2 potatoes chopped
1/2 tsp. garlic powder
1/4 tsp. pepper

Mix ingredients.

Cook in pressure cooker with steady hissing for 35 minutes. Let pressure drop of its own accord. Just before serving add 3 tbsp. lemon juice.[7]

Bowman Black-eyed Pea Stew

Combine in a pot:

1 lb. dried black-eyed peas, prepped*
1/4 head cabbage chopped
1 28-oz. can tomatoes (or fresh equivalent)
3 potatoes cubed
3 carrots diced
1 onion sliced
9 to 10 cups water
2 tsp. salt
1/2 tsp. pepper
3 tbsp. olive oil
1 clove garlic crushed

Add sliced yellow squash and zucchini to make it even nicer.

Simmer for 20 minutes.

Other Legume Recipes

Add a starch and a vegetable to one of the following dishes to serve a nutritionally complete meal.

Black-eyed Peas

Put in saucepan:

1 lb. dried black-eyed peas, prepped*
2 tsp. salt
2 tbsp. oil (we use olive oil)
Can also add sauteed onion and garlic for extra flavor.

Barely cover with water.

Simmer for 15 or 20 minutes and serve over rice or with whole grain bread.

Kidney Beans

Combine in pressure cooker (or slow cooker):

1 lb. dried kidney beans, prepped*
3 tsp. beef bullion
1 28-oz. can tomatoes (or fresh equivalent)
1 chopped onion
1 tbsp. chili powder
1/2 tsp. salt
1 cup TVP (textured vegetable protein) optional

Barely cover with water in pressure cooker (or 4 cups water in slow cooker). Mix ingredients. Cook in pressure cooker 25 minutes with cooker hissing consistently. Let pressure drop of its own accord.

Baked Beans with Molasses

Combine in pressure cooker (or slow cooker):

1 lb. dried Northern beans, prepped*
1/4 lb. diced bacon (or 1/3 cup bacon-flavored TVP)
3 tbsp. brown sugar
3 tbsp. molasses
1 tsp. salt
1/2 tsp. mustard
1 onion chopped
2 tbsp. ketchup

Barely cover with water in pressure cooker (or 4 cups water in slow cooker). Mix ingredients. Cook with steady hissing 45 minutes. Let pressure drop of own accord.[8]

Lentil Stew

Combine:

2 cups lentils (rinsed and sorted)
8 cups water
1 onion chopped
3 carrots chopped
1/3 head cabbage chopped
1 tsp. salt
1/4 tsp. pepper
2 tbsp. olive oil

Simmer approximately 20-30 minutes until lentils are tender. Serve this lentil stew with corn bread or whole wheat bread to make a complete meal.

Note: Some have expressed concern over the use of canned tomatoes due to their possible toxicity. Instead of canned tomatoes, one could substitute fresh ones, ones in glass jars, Tetra Pak boxes, or bottled pasta sauce.

Debra Ridings's Whole Wheat Bread

Grind* 12 cups of whole wheat berries (half Hard Red and half Hard White).

Turn oven to warm and insert dough hook into dough maker.*

Measure 6 cups of flour into dough maker. Add:

2 tbsp. salt
2 tbsp. fresh yeast
1/3 cup gluten
2/3 cup cooking oil
2/3 cup honey
1/3 cup lecithin
1/4 cup ground flaxseed (optional)
6 cups warm water (100°–110°F)

*We use Grain Master Whisper Mill and DLX2000 dough maker by Magic Mill.

Turn mixer on low speed until all ingredients are pretty well blended. Then increase the mixer's speed and add flour by half cupfuls, mixing well after each addition. When the dough starts to clean the side of the bowl, stop adding flour and set the mixer for 8 minutes.

While the dough is kneading, spray four bread pans with non-stick coating. Lightly oil hands and the surface for shaping the loaves. When the dough maker is finished kneading remove the dough, divide and shape it into four loaves.

Place the dough in pans and let it rise in the warm oven until doubled in size (our oven takes 33 minutes). Do not open the oven door once the dough is "proofing" or it will collapse. Check on the loaves using the oven light and window.

Turn the oven temperature to 350° and bake until the loaves sound hollow when tapped on the top (our oven takes 45 minutes).

Butter the tops of the loaves and let them cool in the pans for 10 minutes. Remove the loaves from the pans.[9]

Everything is made good until man makes it bad. He does what tastes good and feels good even if he kills himself in the process.

Hors d'oeuvres, they really save a meal. A hostess doesn't have to cook as much for her guests because hors d'oeuvres kill their appetite. By the time the guests have a few drinks and hors d'oeuvres, the hostess doesn't have to worry about the main meal. It's a trick! It works two ways—it saves food and it wrecks health, thereby helping doctors make a living. I've always enjoyed riding horseback in the mountains. We'd see the pretty rhododendron and mountain laurel. The leaves are a beautiful green; so gorgeous. Why won't that horse just take one bite of those leaves? They're poisonous. No, he wouldn't touch them! He'll eat the grass and the briars. But a man, he'll take just a taste. He'll say, "I just have to have a little of those green leaves."

Routine

Children need the security of routine. There should be regularly scheduled meals, naps, work, play, and bed times. Our Creator designed an orderly universe. Spring always follows winter. Day follows night.[10] Even the animals follow their own instinctive routines.[11] We humans would be wise to follow suit. Our bodies function best on routine, allowing us to be more productive long term.

A routine understood by all members of the household promotes peace. Most children would not object to naps if they came at the same time every day. All the family would be happier and healthier if parents exercised the discipline of eating at regular intervals and going to bed at a sensible hour. Are we *"making straight paths for our feet"*?[12] So many headaches, stomachaches, and short tempers could be avoided simply by eating and sleeping according to a consistent schedule.

Routines aren't etched in stone. Life brings many interruptions and sometimes crises. You can't neglect hospitality if friends drop by at mealtimes. Babies don't become ill on schedule. If, however, a family has developed a basic set of good habits, occasional interruptions won't destroy them. When interruptions and crises pass, order is quickly restored.

It's best to establish household schedules in conjunction with your husband's work schedule. They may have to be tweaked as your family grows and changes.

Dr. Denmark recommended the following:

6:00 a.m.   Wake-up time
7:00 a.m.   Breakfast
9:00 a.m.   Baby's naptime
12:30 p.m. Lunch
6:00 p.m.   Supper, bedtime for baby afterward

At our house we follow an adapted version that works well.

6:00 a.m.	Mom and Dad wake-up time
6:30 a.m.	Children wake up
7:00 a.m.	Breakfast
	Family worship
	Chores
10:00 a.m.–1:00 p.m.	Home schooling and naptime for babies
1:00 p.m.	Lunch; playtime
4:00 p.m.	Prepare supper
6:00 p.m.	Evening chores (everyone)
6:30 p.m.	Supper
7:00 p.m.	Bath and bed for young children
9:00–10:00 p.m.	Bed for older children (Eighteen years old and up establish their own bedtime.)

Sleep

It is vain for you to rise up early. To retire late. To eat the bread of painful labors; For He gives to His beloved even in his sleep.[13]

The Creator has told us we need rest. We need to rest on Sunday and maintain good sleeping habits. If our bodies don't get sufficient rest, there are inevitable consequences: fatigue, depression, short temper, increased susceptibility to illness, discouragement, anxiety. The list could continue. When the prophet Elijah was afraid and discouraged, God dealt with his exhaustion before he encouraged and instructed him verbally.[14]

Children grow in their sleep and require plenty of undisturbed rest to realize their full growth potential. Without it, they will be unable to learn properly during waking hours. As always, maintain a balance. Some people have a tendency to sleep too long. Individual sleep requirements vary, so be sensitive to your children's particular needs.

Average Sleep Requirements

Newborn:	20 hours
3 months:	16 hours
2 years:	12 hours
6 years:	12 hours
Adolescent:	8 hours
Adult:	8 hours

Teenage children need more sleep than they are getting today. Good sleeping habits have to start from birth and as the child grows older, he should not be tempted by things in the home or outside attractions. Children today old enough to be interested in radio, television, [computer games, Internet], movies, scouting, clubs of many kinds, or sports have little or no chance to get the required amount of sleep. They see their parents doing without sleep and they feel like they [shouldn't] be told they need sleep.

We parents may say we don't need sleep anymore, but that is not a true statement. Every person who expects his or her body to function its best must have sleep, at night if possible, and it should be at least eight hours. We may never go back to the idea that night was made for rest, as we have the excitement of night to attract us, but parents should teach their children the value of sleep if they are to get out of their bodies the best that is there.[15]

Sometimes I'm tempted to think Thomas Edison did our family a disservice. It must have been much easier for everyone to get necessary sleep before electric lights were invented!

When Dr. Denmark was a child, she remembered her mother lighting a big lamp after supper dishes were cleared. She set the lamp in the middle of their long table, then helped all the children with homework. After lessons were learned, out went the lamp and children to bed.

In early years, all my little ones were tucked into bed shortly after supper. Now that they are older, our evenings are quite different. Most chores and schoolwork have been completed, so after supper the "party" begins: conversation, laughter, stories, and music into the night. It's fun, but I try to be mindful that all of us (especially John and Emily) still need adequate rest. The advent of light bulbs didn't eliminate necessity of sleep.

Sunshine and Exercise

Encourage your children to play outdoors. When an infant is two weeks old, take him out in the sun for five to ten minutes daily. But as we all know, overexposure to the sun's rays is harmful to the skin. Be sensible and don't allow your children to overdo it. Dr. Denmark recommended covering them with hats and clothing rather than using a sunscreen.

When I came to Atlanta in 1928, there were innumerable cases of rickets due to the sheet of smoke that covered the city. The trains puffed and furnaces burned soft coal. People kept house lights on and had mustaches by 10:00 a.m. Kids' arms and legs were bowed. They were obtaining plenty of calcium from evaporated milk but had rickets because their skin lacked exposure to sunshine. People, especially fair-skinned individuals, should never bake in the sun. We do, however, need a certain amount of sunshine for vitamin D.

Encourage exercise by providing a few basic toys like balls, jump ropes, bicycles, or skates. Given the opportunity, most healthy children will get all the exercise they need on their own. Some, however, tend to be sedentary and need more stimulation. Parents can be creative in motivating inactive children, possibly with an outdoor playhouse, exercising a pet, or taking soccer lessons. **Take care not to allow children's sports to dominate your family life.**

Guarding Our Children's Health

In the days before immunizations and antibiotics, infant mortality was 162.4 per thousand births (1900).[16] My great-grandmother lived with constant concern for her infant's health. Letters she wrote to her mother reveal her vigilance in protecting him. She shielded him from chills, was anxious that he receive enough fresh air and sunshine, and guarded against germs. She paid particular attention to what he ate and saw that he had plenty of sleep. If her son was ever ill, she was meticulously careful in nursing him back to full recovery. The stakes were too high not to be careful. Serious diseases were commonplace, and so were infant tombstones.

With the advent of modern medicine, infant mortality dropped to 8.9 per thousand births by 1991.[17] What a miracle! But mothers have become complacent and are no longer as conscientious as their predecessors were. That youngsters get adequate rest, nourishment, sunshine, and nursing care isn't a priority in many homes, yet such laxness is detrimental to their long-term health. To reach their full potential physically and mentally, children must build sturdy bodies through good health habits—bodies that last far beyond childhood into ripe old age.

Infants and young children grow at an enormous rate, and sickness interrupts their growth. When they become ill, let's nurse them to full recovery before dragging them out in public. Let them stay home and rest, be quiet, have a chance to heal.

Is your child sick with a fever? Give him a warm bath, fresh pajamas. Change the sheets on his bed. Give him a special book or game to play with, but be sure he rests. He should be fever-free for two evenings before resuming normal activities. It's best for him and for the other children who are exposed to him. When recovering from an intestinal problem, he should have easily digestible food for a few days. A child getting over the flu should stay out of public for one week to allow his immunities to rebuild.

Illness can draw a family together, offer opportunity to show love for your child, and increase his sense of security. Remember we are building bodies for the future.

I think with gratitude of the excellent nursing care I received from my mother when I was sick. There were hot baths, clean sheets, quietness, good food, and cheerful words. Certainly I despised medicine, needles, and other discomforts and protested them vigorously. Down inside, though, I knew they were in my best interest. There was a wonderful comfort in knowing I was well cared for.

The most important factors in keeping children healthy are a good diet, a good schedule, and keeping them away from sick children.

Notes

1. Leila Daughtry-Denmark, M.D., *Every Child Should Have a Chance* (Atlanta, GA: 1971), 214

2. Denmark, *Every Child Should Have a Chance*, 41

3. Denmark, *Every Child Should Have a Chance*, 72

4. *Rival Crock Pot Cookbook*, 16

5. Gloria Repp, *Noodle Soup* (Greenville, SC: BJU Press 1994), 28-29

6. Doris Janzen Longacre, *More-With-Less Cookbook* (Scottdale, PA: Herald Press, 1988), 137

7. Recipe on back of Jack Rabbit *Black Turtle Beans.*

8. *Presto Pressure Cooker* (Eau Claire, WI: Johnson Printing, Inc., 1979),51

9. Debra Ridings, *Feeding the Shepherd's Flocks* (Kearney, NE: Morris Press 1999), 6

10. Genesis 8:22

11. Psalm 104:19-30

12. Hebrews 12:13

13. Psalm 127:2

14. 1 Kings 19:3–18

15. Denmark, *Every Child Should Have a Chance*, 157

16. Historical Statistics of the United States: Colonial Times to 1970 (Washington, D.C.: Government Printing Office, 1975)

17. *Statistical Abstracts of the United States* (Washington, D.C.: U.S. Department of Commerce, 1994).

𝕤 12 𝕢
What is Needful?

It was Monday. One glance at the calendar filled me with dread! What a schedule for the week: doctors' appointments, piano lessons, evening meetings, rehearsals, and a birthday party. The joy of Sunday worship quickly disappeared.

When the children saw me looking at the calendar they surmised it was time to push their particular agendas. A chorus of voices rang out.

"I need a new pair of tennis shoes. Can we go shopping today?"

"Can Rebekah spend the night Friday?"

"You promised to take us to the lake; when are we going?"

Something snapped. "Be quiet!" I barked. "Go back to your rooms and get your chores done—now!" Dead silence and hurt looks. "Dear Jesus," I breathed, "forgive my short temper. The needs of my children are overwhelming and I am so burdened. Please help me." At that moment Scripture came to mind and chided my turbulent spirit.

"Martha, Martha, you are worried and bothered about so many things; but only one thing is needful, for Mary has chosen the good part, which shall not be taken away from her." [1] *"Seek first His kingdom and His righteousness, and all these things shall be added to you."* [2]

We must evaluate our priorities. Even good possessions and wholesome activities may not be important at the moment.

Charles E. Hummel wisely wrote: "It is not God who loads us until we bend or crack with an ulcer, nervous breakdown, heart attack, or stroke. These come from our inner compulsions, coupled with the pressure of circumstances." He warns against "letting the urgent things crowd out the important."[3] I often have to remind myself of the fact that **God gives His children sufficient time and strength to accomplish the work He has intended for their lives each and every new day.**

Martha of Bethany was frantically busy with what she perceived as important work while Mary sat at Jesus' feet listening and learning from Him. Mary had discerned what was important for that moment and was commended for it. Think about Jesus' words and Mary's example. Midst the frenzy of everyday life, are we doing what matters?

Consistent with our entertatinment-obsessed age, there are those who treat children like toys, spoiling and delighting in them for a time, but neglectful when the novelty of parenting wanes or life becomes challenging. Unquestionably, children can be amusing. Nonetheless, they are definitely not entrusted to us for yet another diversion or source of personal enrichment. They are living souls and rearing them is a sacred stewardship. Parents, in chasing our desires, are we neglecting our children? In attempting to satisfy their wants, are we losing sight of their true needs?

Other than a child's need for health and his mother's presence, what is critical for him? Most children in our culture are amply supplied any indulgence money can buy. Yet so many important essentials are neglected which require gifts of time, love, and discipline.

The following discussion is not intended to be exhaustive, nor do I claim to be an ultimate authority on the subject. However, as Dr. Denmark encouraged me, I would like to encourage every mom who reads this book to periodically reevaluate her own priorities and thoughtfully determine the individual needs of her children. It's usually best to avoid either comparing one's family with the neighbor's or consulting your child's desires. Instead, study him with a prayer for wisdom, look to scriptural principles to guide you in determining what is crucial to his well-being, and commit to being a responsible mother. One cannot be a loving mother apart from being a responsible one.

Isn't the essence of mothering to discern the true needs of our offspring and give of ourselves sacrificially to meet them? Furthermore, could it be that while mothering we might discover our own true needs along the way?

My father had a wonderful way of responding to our requests when we asked for something. He'd suggest we study it for three weeks, then see whether we still wanted the item. Nine times out of ten, we lost interest. I think about some of the boys I used to like. Oh, they were great, but what if I had married one of them? It would have wrecked my life! What if God gave us everything we prayed for? Some things we desire may not be good for us. We can't have everything we want.

Patience, patience, patience…a mother needs to be so patient and to be a real diplomat, too. Everyone gives her advice (adults and children alike). She should listen carefully, respectfully, to it all and then just do what she thinks is best.

Obedience

One of the most fundamental needs a child has is training in obedience. He needs to learn at a very early age to obey the God-ordained authorities in his life. An obedient child is typically happier, less frustrated, more self-controlled, and more likely to follow the commands of God as he grows in maturity. Obedient children are a joy to be around.

It is not within the scope of this chapter to address obedience training in detail. However, a few basic principles will be touched on:

Parents should be confident in their authority because it is delegated authority from God himself. *"Children, obey your parents in the Lord, for this is right. Honor your father and mother (which is the first commandment with a promise), so that it may be well with you, and that you may live long on the earth."*[4]

Certainly there are limits to any human authority; a parent must never use psychological or physical abuse during the training process, nor require children to do something unethical. On the other hand, parents need never feel apologetic about assuming a firm, authoritative role, or worry that insisting on compliance will somehow damage their child's psyche, ability to mature and make decisions. Instead, a loving, confident, consistent, controlled exercise of parental authority builds a sense of security and maturity. It also fosters a peaceful home!

Children should be required to obey quickly and cheerfully. It is a mistake to attempt to reason or persuade a young child into obedience. "Little people" do not possess mature reasoning skills. Nor is it appropriate to assume the position of an attorney arguing before a judge (the child). Attempting to reason a child into compliance is not maintaining one's authority. It is putting the child into the position of authority and can foster pride.

Jerry White, a wise educator/pastor/counselor once wrote, "…if you have to tell your children repeatedly to do anything, often times having to get 'stern' before you get the right and desired response, then be honest about the fact that they are not obeying you. Obedience on their terms is disobedience and manifests a heart of rebellion against your authority. Teach and demand respect and obedience, basically without question if you want to have a secure child. This obviously is assuming that you are teaching and establishing rules of conduct and speech based on Truth (II Timothy 3:14-17; Psalm 19:7-11; 119:9). In doing this, you prepare and equip your children to receive and grasp the principles of God's truth…

"As a parent, recognize that teaching (giving instruction) without training (demanding compliance with and obedience to that which is taught) equals an exercise in futility destined for failure before it starts for you and your child, the result of which will be frustration for you and frustration plus increasing insecurity for your child as he or she grows and matures developmentally. Failure to see and recognize this is one way a father, and mother secondarily, can be provoking their children to anger. God's word is not unclear—Ephesians 6:1-4. To '*bring them up in the nurture and admonition of the Lord*' is to demand that they learn, at an early age (6 months) to obey you whether they understand why you require what you do or not. What you require should primarily be obedience as determined by the principles of God's word, and your child/children should be expected and made to obey—period, with or without understanding—Proverbs 3:4-6 is a principle involved here."[5]

Note: After young people have gained maturity and demonstrated respectful obedience towards their parents, it is certainly appropriate and important to discuss with them the reasons behind requirements. For further guidance on obedience training, refer to a recommended list of resources on page 228.

Teaching a child what love means is a painful process at times. We must see our child want things that are not good and not have them, and we must see him punished for misdeeds and not apologize for the punishment. Love never gives over to persuasion if it is not good for the child. The insecure child is one who knows he can get what he wants by crying or a temper tantrum.[6]

[If a little child is trying to help mother in the kitchen and accidently breaks her best cup], she should not raise her voice or punish him, but tell him that was mama's best cup, and now it is gone, and we can't have it any more. She should tell him when he helps her, to hold things tight so they will not drop. Then he will learn a lesson and not be discouraged in his efforts.

If this same little boy picked up a cup in a temper and threw it across the room, the good old tried-and-proven method of discipline should be used. A little switch to the legs is the best method, and his mother should not say she is sorry she switched him. We punish a child because we love him and want him to have the right training... This matter of rearing children is the most tedious, demanding job on earth, and there is no substitute for a mother.[7]

A Good Teacher

Jesus Christ was the consummate teacher of all time. He taught by word and deed, in truth and love. He did not instruct his disciples in a four-walled classroom or assign them a stack of text-books to read (although classrooms and books have their limited place). He taught them by showing them a way of life, instructing them as they lived together, perfectly fulfilling the directives of Deuteronomy 6:4-9:

"Hear O Israel! The Lord our God, the Lord is one! You shall love the Lord your God with all your heart and with all your soul and with all your might. These words which I am commanding you today shall be on your heart. You shall teach them diligently to your sons and shall talk of them when you sit in your house and when you walk by the way and when you lie down and when you rise up. You shall bind them as a sign on your hand and they shall be as frontals on your forehead. You shall write them on the door posts of your house and on your gates."

Follow Christ's example, and model for your children an excellent way of life, teaching them as you live together. Our current culture is infected by chaotic, dissipated, hypercasual, and self-centered living. Our children have plenty of examples of how **not** to live. Smiling celebrities abound at every check-out line and on every computer/TV screen. Teach your children the truth—that these siren smiles belie miserable and shipwrecked lives.

Show your children how and why they must turn away from prevailing cultural norms and at times be willing to stand alone for truth. Instruct your children as you meet challenges, make decisions, sit at the dinner table, drive places, make purchases, celebrate success, face disappointments, as you work and play.

Show them by example how to live a disciplined life, how to dress with dignity and how to interact courteously with others. Model good table manners, health habits, and lives of service to God and man.

Consideration of others does not come naturally, nor strictly by good example. Children require careful, verbal instruction on how to show courtesy to strangers, friends, and authorities (including parents).

It's best to seize teachable moments. Your children are more likely to learn if they have asked a question and expressed interest in a particular subject. Jesus even turned a rivalry between His disciples into a teaching opportunity.[8]

None of us is perfect. Be honest about your inconsistencies. When you fail, ask your children to forgive you and pray for you. Most children are quick to forgive if parents are honest and humble.

We hear so much today about parents getting down on a level with their children. Our children don't want us parents to get down on their level. They want us to be adults and somebody they can look up to. A child has other children his age to play the game of life with, and wants his parents to be examples of perfect adults. If a little girl wants to play lady, she uses her mother as an example. That mother should be the example she wants her daughter to be... Many women are not what they want their daughters to be, so the daughter never gets to play lady, for her mother is not a lady. In too many instances mother dresses, talks, fights, argues, and behaves like a child.[9]

Once a man asked me to "straighten out" his three wayward children. The mother's teeth were so brown from tobacco stains that when she smiled her mouth looked like a dark hole. The father looked even worse. I thought to myself, "If I had a stallion that looked like that man and a mare that looked like that mother, I wouldn't expect their colt to be a Kentucky race horse!"

Many children possess a beguiling sense of confidence in their own discretion. They are certain they know what they need and what's best for them. If you're at all insecure in your own judgment, their confident assertions can easily sway you. Children are masters at lobbying for their own agendas. In truth, children have very little discernment as to what is best for them. Did your ten-year-old really have to stay up until midnight? Did Suzie need that bag of candy? Is it really imperative that your teenager attend that gathering?

Parents shouldn't allow themselves to be guilt-manipulated by their children or by other parents. Parents, guided by God's Word, ought to be the source of direction. "This food is what's best for your body...That activity is bad for your spiritual growth...No, we are not going to watch that movie." Your children need your direction and example far more than they may ever admit.

Suppose someone brought a stranger to Atlanta, letting him off at Five Points with no maps or directions, and told him to find his way home. Which road would he take? There are a dozen intersections there offering a hundred ways he might go.

If a child knows where home is, he'll know how to live. My mother kept me home for eight years before I went to school. I was a Daughtry. I knew the Daughtry way of life; I knew the way home. Had my early childhood been spent in a day-care center, I would have seen many different ways of life. A little fellow in day-care is in the middle of the city and doesn't know how to get home.

Papa

The marriage relationship was intended to reflect Christ's relationship with His Church.[10] One of the greatest opportunities we have to testify of Christ, is to be a faithful spouse, reflecting that divine relationship to our neighbors and children. Mothers, try to model submission and respect in your relationship with your husband. When your children observe your patient and respectful attitude, it will be much easier for them to respond that way to you.

Nurture your relationship with your spouse. Your child will never have more than one father. No one can ever replace his Papa. Conversation between parents should be congenial and characterized by mutual respect. Remember, mothers, your husband has just as much a right to his opinion as you do to yours.

Not once do I recall my parents arguing with one another. The harmony in their relationship created a sense of security and well-being in our home. By watching them we learned to get along with each other.

A mother should do the best she can with what she has to create a pleasant home environment for Papa and the kids. A woman came into my office one day at the Central Presbyterian Clinic where I used to volunteer. She lived in the slums, was ragged, dirty with tobacco stains at the corners of her mouth. Her two little girls looked like she did except for the tobacco. She told me, "Dr. Denmark, I'm so worried. My man isn't coming home regularly anymore. I'm sure he's drinking and misbehaving." After one good look at her I could see why he didn't want to come home.

Instead of giving her supplies (the clinic had those available), it seemed best to help her change her lifestyle. "Mrs. Jones," I said. "Let's try a plan for two months. You go home and get some soap. Clean the house, and you and your daughters bathe. Curl your and your little girl's hair. Put a nice clean cloth or even some clean paper (whatever is available) on the table. Then serve whatever you have and make it as tasty as you can. Serve three meals a day and clean up after each one. Let's try this plan for two months and see what happens." After two months she came back elated with good news. "Dr. Denmark, I've never seen a man change so much in all my life!"

Back to the Basics

When Scripture promises *"God shall supply all your needs according to His riches in glory in Christ Jesus,"*[11] I don't believe it necessarily refers to a new car or a steak every Friday night. When addressing physical needs, it generally speaks of essentials in terms of food, clothing, and shelter.

There was a time when women took pride in doing a good job with the basics—clean clothes, a clean house, and nourishing food. We should find joy in the same.

Are you so busy with the extracurricular that your children live on fast or convenience foods. Are their sheets clean? Are they learning how to keep their rooms neat? Is your little girl's hair well brushed. Does your son need a haircut? Is your newborn getting enough quiet time? Even more important—are you reading the Bible and praying together?

Some are more capable than others of juggling numerous activities while furnishing the basics. You must realistically evaluate your own capabilities and responsibilities and be at peace with the measure God has provided you. Finances, energy level, organizational skills, number and ages of children, husband's support, and many other factors influence whether we are a "one- or five-ring-circus" mom.

If the basics are sliding, you may need to eliminate other commitments. It's vital to the tranquility of your home that you be content. Successfully managing family responsibilities is an accomplishment that shouldn't be minimized. All who do it deserve congratulations and encouragement. How quickly life can become chaotic and marriages strained when a mother is unable to handle her primary duties. I advise moms, especially those with young children, to be extremely hesitant about committing themselves to outside activities. If they want to do a good job at home, it's wise for them to minimize time spent in the car, on the Internet, and in trivial conversations on the phone. Do I have to mention switching off the TV?

When a child is reared in an environment of confusion and uncertainty—without a system and good planning—the chances that he will find a happy, meaningful, and productive way of life are lessened. A child who is reared in a jumble cannot think as clearly as a child who is reared in a home where there is order, cleanliness, and a good system… The keeping of the house means the keeping of a life.[12]

My philosophy is that if a mother runs her house like a man runs a good business, it will be a success. Building a child is the biggest business on earth.[13]

Time

Our generation has forgotten how to live. Trying desperately to grab the most out of life, many of us have thrown our lives away. We drag our children along at our frantic pace, anxious that they receive the best of all possible educational and social experiences.

Don't forget that children, particularly very young children, need time to ponder, to observe nature, and relax. Curling up in a corner with a book, eating and digesting food, asking questions of an attentive listener—all enhance their daily growth and take time. Slow down, mothers. Learn to enjoy simple pleasures like taking the kids for a walk in the neighborhood. Read them a good story. Let them help or just watch while you make a special Friday- night dessert. Don't get stuck on the treadmill of overcommitting your finances or your time (a much more valuable commodity). In both cases it's enormously stressful. I write from personal experience. Keep in mind that investing unhurried time in the lives of your little ones will bring far greater returns than any monetary investment you can make.

I don't remember my mother ever being in a hurry or raising her voice at any one of us. She never made us feel we were working her to death, and I never heard her say, "You children are wearing me out!"

How did she stay so patient with 12 children? I think if you had been in my office today, you'd wonder how I stay so calm. There were babies crying in both side rooms, mamas slapping and yelling. I could get awfully upset. I could lose my temper at the parents and say, "Don't come back if you won't follow my advice."

I think my mother handled it just the way I do; she had self control. If you don't have it, you'd better find some. If a mother raises her voice, the children will too. If she slaps, they will follow her example. Sometimes I'm asked, "Dr. Denmark, what makes my children so bad?"

"Go look in the mirror," I say, "You get apples off apple trees."

In contrast to our frenzied existence stands the example of Christ. Charles Hummel observes: "His life was never feverish; He had time for people. He could spend hours talking to one person, such as the Samaritan woman at the well. His life showed wonderful balance…"14

Excessive outside activities can actually promote dissatisfaction. We have found that limiting activities causes our children to be more content with home life, and more likely to enjoy and appreciate the time they get to do something special.

Moms are often so busy driving their children from place to place that they neglect critical training. There is no time to address bad attitudes, insist on neatness, or teach children to be kind to each other. Mom is too distracted with rushing everyone off to the next event.

If a little one says he's bored, don't assume he needs additional stimulation from outside activities and/or sophisticated toys. Certainly don't turn on the television or computer games. Video games and TV tend to sap his creative energies, shorten attention span, and make him feel wired or discontent. Instead, hand him some art supplies, seeds to plant, or building toys. Give him a roll of masking tape and a cardboard box. A blanket and chairs make a great tent. Restlessness can be an excellent stimulus for creativity and productivity.

Extracurricular activities are great, but they shouldn't interfere with family relationships. I'm all for sports, but many children involved in them don't eat supper with the family. I knew one little girl whose activities almost wrecked her. She was taking violin, organ, and dancing lessons. That child never had a chance to play or have quiet times at home. She never had time to go into her room and be creative.

Everybody has time to do the things he wants to do. We need to psychoanalyze ourselves, asking, "Is it that I don't have the time or that I don't want to take the time?" Anything we have to do is work. Anything we want to do is play.

Adolescents and Time

As much as young children need time for quietness, reflection, and creativity, so older children in the midst of hormonal changes need to be busy. Idleness is surely the devil's workshop when it comes to adolescents. Bad behavior during the teen years can cause permanent damage to a child's future. Much depression, frustration, immorality, and unhealthy introspection may be avoided if young adults are occupied with plenty of wholesome activities.

Busyness doesn't have to be hectic, but keep your young adults occupied with chores, challenging projects, community service, inspiring books, or a family business. Help them follow their own positive interests and discover their individual strengths and weaknesses through work and responsibility.

Do not fail to take lots of time to talk to your adolescent children. This can hardly be stressed too much. It is critical that you have a glimpse into their hearts and know what they are thinking. Also, it is vital that they understand why you believe the things you do and hold to the standards you have. Talk over experiences, relationships, studies, current events, feelings, aspirations, struggles, sermons, and everything that is important to them.

The adolescent years are like those of a woman going through menopause. There are a lot of hormonal changes, but you have to go through it. If a woman can keep very busy during that period, leave off taking estrogen and all that mess women typically take during those changes, and stay out of doctors' offices, she would be better off. Eventually menopause will pass and she can settle down to being a nice old lady. When adolescents pass through their hormonal changes, they begin to settle down too.

There is no guarantee a child will turn out right no matter how wonderful his parents have been or excellent his upbringing. There comes a time when he must make his own choices. However, if he has been brought up right he has had a model to follow. He knows right from wrong and…I do believe the prodigal son came back because he remembered those clean, white sheets and that good fried chicken!

Jacob Abbott's Wisdom

Jacob Abbott's book *Training Children in Godliness* was so helpful to me in evaluating priorities and planning my work that I have quoted a number of paragraphs from the chapter entitled "Teaching Children to Be Happy." The words of this nineteenth-century educator, minister, and author will never grow outdated.

"So whatever may be the reader's situation and condition in life, if he wishes to be happy, let him regulate his affairs. If you have uncertain, unsettled accounts open, which you have been dreading to examine, go and explore the cases thoroughly and have them closed. If there are plans which you have been intending to accomplish, but which you have been postponing, summon your resolution and carry them at once into effect, or else determine to abandon them and dismiss them from your thoughts.

"The mind of young and ardent man becomes loaded with crude, half-formed designs, unfinished plans, and duties postponed. He is like a child unaccustomed to the world, who takes a walk on a pleasant summer's day. Every object seems valuable, and he picks up a pebble here, a stick there, and gathers a load of pretty flowers in this place and that, until he becomes so encumbered with his treasures that he can hardly go on. They are constantly slipping and dropping from his hands, and become a source of perplexity and anxiety to him because he cannot retain them all. So it is with us. Every plan which reason forms or imagination paints, we think we must execute; but after having made a new beginning, a new project which we are equally eager to secure enters our heads. In a short time, we become encumbered with a mass of intellectual lumber which we cannot carry and are unwilling to leave. Consider what you can and will execute, and take hold of the execution of them now. Abandon the rest, so that you may move forward with a mind that is free and uncluttered.

"This, then, is the second great rule for securing personal happiness. Look over your affairs, and arrange and methodize everything. Define in your own mind what you have to do, and dismiss everything else. Take time for reflection, and plan all your work so as to go on smoothly and quietly so that the mind may be ahead of all its duties, choosing its own way, and going forward in peace.

"There is one point in connection with this subject of the management of worldly affairs which should not be passed by, and which is yet an indispensable condition of human happiness. I mean the duty of every man to bring his expenses and his financial liabilities fairly within his control. There are some cases of a peculiar character, and some occasional emergencies, perhaps, in the life of every person, which constitute exceptions; but this is the general rule.

"Reduce your expenditures, your style of living, and your business far below your financial means, so that you may have money in plenty.... Almost all are eagerly reaching forward to a station in life a little above what they can well afford, or struggling to do a business a little more extensive than they have capital or steady credit for. Thus, all through life they keep just above their means; and just above, by even a small excess, is inevitable misery.

"If your aim is happiness, reduce your style of living and your responsibilities of business to such a point that you shall easily be able to reach it. Do this, I say, at all costs... For there is such a thing as happiness in a single room, with plain furniture and simple fare; but there is no such thing as happiness, with responsibilities which cannot be met and debts increasing, without any prospect of their discharge. If your object is power, the credit of belonging to good society, or the most rapid accumulation of property, and you are willing to sacrifice happiness for it, I might perhaps give you different advice. But if your object is happiness, then this is the only way."[15]

If parents would just teach their children that everything has a price. One of the most important phrases for them to learn is "I can't afford it." I'll never forget what Mary said one day to a friend as they played outside my window. She was admiring the other child's pretty dress.

"Why don't you ask your mother to buy you one like it?" the little girl asked.

"We can't afford it," Mary answered. I was so glad to hear her say that. She learned as a child that there were things we couldn't afford, and she was content with what she had. I've never heard her complain about not having enough.

Friendships

I have spoken to scores of mothers who voice deep concern over the social development of their children. Moms are often advised that even toddlers need to spend lots of time in group settings with peers. Ostensibly, if children do not participate in mother's morning out programs, preschool sports, and day-care settings, they will never learn to cope with life's challenges, make friends, or be independent thinkers.

I am convinced that the reverse is true. Young children who have not been abandoned to the company of peers, who feel secure in the care and love of their parents, are far more likely to develop social confidence and be able to form fast friendships.

Time spent with peers at an early age is far overrated. Children are more likely to learn bad behavior from other children than good behavior. In my experience, the more time my children spent with their peers during formative years, the more trouble I had with their attitudes. This is one of the many reasons we chose to home educate.

Certainly there is a place for friendships outside the home, but children are far more likely to learn good social skills from their parents. Model courtesy, kindness, patience, and thoughtfulness for your children. The best training for friendships begins in the home between family members. Good relationships between siblings can translate to good friendships outside the home. Encourage brothers and sisters to be best friends.

Encourage your children to make distinctions between degrees of intimacy, being careful not to share their inmost thoughts with strangers in person or on Facebook. Author Harvey Newcomb, is wise when he writes the following:

"You may be courteous and polite to all, wherever and whenever you meet them, and yet maintain such a prudent reserve, and cautious deportment as not to be much exposed to contamination, if they should not prove suitable companions. But everyone needs intimate friends; and it is necessary that these should be well chosen. A bad friend may prove your ruin. You should therefore be slow and cautious in the formation of intimacies and friendships. Do not be suddenly taken with anyone, and so enter into a hasty friendship; for you may be mistaken and soon repent of it. There is much force in the old adage, 'All is not gold that shines.' A pleasing exterior often conceals a corrupt heart. Before you enter into close intimacies or friendships, study the characters of the persons whom you propose to choose for companions."[16]

Teach your children to be kind and polite to everyone, but not choose close friends with those who are immoral, hot-tempered, or gossipy. If an individual gossips with you about others, it is likely they will talk about you in your absence and cannot be trusted to keep confidences.

Friendships are important but shouldn't take up all of our time. The Scriptures warn against becoming a busybody.[17] It's easy to be a busybody when excessive time is spent social networking. Our friendships should encourage us to *"love and good deeds."*[18] We need to avoid wasting time on the Internet and gossiping when efforts should be devoted to meaningful work.

If your child wants good friends, stress that he needs to **be** a good friend. It's important to be polite, keep confidences, show interest in others, ask questions, and be willing to quickly overlook minor offenses.

Friendships between sexes should be characterized by the same qualities of kindness, respect, and purity. Young people need to be reminded that the young man or woman they are associating with is someone's child and will likely be someone's spouse. Would that young man or young woman's parents or future spouse appreciate the way they are being treated? Young people should treat those of the opposite sex how they would want their future spouse to be treated.

Boys should be taught that all girls should have the love and respect that they would want for their own mothers, sisters, or daughters, and that every girl, no matter how bad she is, is somebody's child. They should be taught that God will punish a man for breaking a law with the lowest type of womanhood as much as he would with the highest type. If she has no character, the sin is no less.[19]

A girl should be taught that a boy or a man will always respect and honor a lady if he is mentally normal or not under the influence of something that causes him to be unable to exercise self-control [such as alcohol]. Good women make good men and a good world. Bad women make bad men and a bad world.[20]

Sometimes adolescents talk with me, bemoaning the fact that a person they have been romantically interested in has taken up with someone else. I always say, "Be glad for them that they found someone. Be happy for them. Besides, it's likely another streetcar will come around the corner soon!"

Romantic relationships need parental involvement and supervision. It is healthiest if friendships are developed in the context of families getting together, instead of age-segregated social groups. Chaperones are still a wise idea. Daytime social gatherings tend to be more conducive to wholesome conversation and interaction rather than late night events when fatigue and excitement loosen control over tongues and behavior. We prefer our young adults to interact with their peers in the context of productive activity (such as service projects or choir practice) rather than simply "hanging out."

In reference to social gatherings, I would like to quote the insightful words of my great-great-grandfather, Reverend Thomas Dwight Witherspoon.

"How many are there, when their children are invited to a place of amusement, or to a social gathering, stop to ask themselves the question, 'What influence will this probably have on their religious character? Will their associates be religious, or irreligious? Will the amusements be such as are baleful to piety and to interest in religious things?'[21]... In how many cases is everything made to bend, not to the religious welfare of the child, but to its position in a fashionable, worldly-minded, and sinful society.[22]

"Can there be any wonder that the child, thus thrown into the midst of irreligious companionships and associations; taught from its earliest childhood that its first duty is to prepare itself to move well in society; that if society is worldly it must be worldly; if society is extravagant, it must be extravagant, if society dissipates, it must dissipate; that it must seek first the good opinion of society, and then, in subordination to that, the kingdom of God: can there be any wonder, I say, that the child is not converted to God? On the other hand, would it not be a very great wonder if, under such circumstances, the child should have any serious impressions at all?[23]

"It is very easy to anticipate the reply that many will make to this. They will meet us with the old trite saying, 'Young people will be young people; they must have some kind of amusement, and you cannot apply the same rules to them that you do to grown people.'

"This is all true enough; but in this very fact that 'young people will be young people,' is found the very strongest argument against the kind of amusements for which this class of persons would plead. Young people not only must have amusement—they will have it. Their nature is joyous; its activities are spontaneous. They will have sport of some kind. If you deny them amusement in one form, they will seek it in another. If you refuse them that which is unwholesome, they will turn to that which is wholesome.[24] [If they are involved in unwholesome amusement]...they will lose all relish for pure and less stimulating pleasures. But keep them away from these, and before you lies a broad field of innocent sports and diversions, from which you may select at will, with the assurance that, together with amusement and recreation, your child may secure health, energy, vigor, and purity.

"But the parent is, perhaps, ready to say further, 'Others send their children to these places of amusement, and mine must go, or be debarred from society.' And who are these others? Christian parents like yourself; excusing themselves on the ground that you, and others like you, allow your children these indulgences. Thus, while you are striving to shift your responsibility on them, they are seeking to rest theirs on you. You are mutually upholding one another in a course which is inconsistent with your covenant vows, in direct violation of the rules of the Church, and in the highest degree destructive of the spiritual interest of your children."[25]

After reading my great-great grandfather's words, I was further convicted that parents with high standards should band together to encourage each other to reject the unwholesome recreation our society offers children. Such parents should provide ample opportunities for wholesome, joyous diversions that will strengthen their children physically and spiritually (see Appendix II).

Clothing

It is true that "clothing does not make a man." However, what we wear is certainly a reflection of who we are, and how we dress our children will influence their behavior. How they learn to dress will also have a great impact on how they are perceived by society. It is vitally important for parents to model for their children appropriate clothing habits. A mother's clothing should be clean, neat, modest, dignified, and feminine. Children will learn from the way she is dressed, and it's important that they not be ashamed of her appearance.

Emphasize to your children the need to dress up more for occasions such as church, weddings, concerts, etc. Formal attire shows respect and usually encourages more "civilized behavior."

The mother of a newborn need only select clothes for her baby that are clean and comfortable. It won't be long, however, before her child will begin to become aware of his gender distinction and should be dressed accordingly. Nurture those God-given feminine and masculine tendencies.

Teach your daughters to dress attractively, but treasure their purity by dressing modestly. Plunging necklines, paper thin or spandex-tight fabrics, thigh-revealing shorts and skirts are carefully utilized by clothing designers to create a sexually alluring look. What about effeminate-looking styles for men or the droopy pants which reveal a young man's backside or boxers? Clothing distributors take advantage of the younger child's desire to feel grownup by offering these styles to progressively younger children.

Parents, do we really want our girls to look like…well, prostitutes…or do we want them to look innocent and attractive? How a young woman dresses reflects her heart and affects her behavior, not to mention how she is treated.

I would like to challenge parents to consciously take charge of the clothing standards in their home and not to give in to the mores of clothing manufacturers. Come up with a written policy of clothing guidelines for your family. Start young if you can, and be very specific. It might mean having to order clothing via the Internet or sewing your own.

Be sensitive to your child's desire to be fashionable. However, if fashionable means trashy and extravagant, garner some resolve. There are times when parents must be kind, but absolutely firm. In my mind, I call those "akimbo times."

Children are going to act the way they are dressed. [Children will emulate the adults they are dressed like.] We can watch little girls at play. They will get a low-necked, tight-fitting, black dress and in a few minutes they are using sticks for cigarettes and something they can find that will represent a cocktail. They are very wicked in their little minds. They will sit with their legs crossed so they can expose as much of their legs as possible, and puff and drink with the greatest glee. Then let these same little girls get into their mothers' house dresses and aprons and they will start making mud pies and playing house.[26]

We must teach our children how to dress. We must teach our daughters that to be beautiful is a gift of God, but to be vulgar is destruction. A girl should be taught that the body should be dressed as beautifully as possible, but she must not accentuate the parts that would tempt a man beyond his self-control.[27]

Every man should dress himself in such a manner as to make his sons and daughters proud of him. A well-dressed man is always handsome, but to see a father going around with his body naked to the waist is not a beautiful sight![28]

Our older sons were thrilled when John was born. After three sisters, finally a rambunctious little brother arrived.

Esther wanted to play with him, too. In fact, in her eyes he was just a big baby doll. She loved to orchestrate events, and it was convenient to have him around because toddler John was the only boy willing to participate in her plays and mock weddings.

Big brothers came home one day to discover John taking part in one of Esther's weddings. The little groom stood dutifully next to a golden-haired bride twice his size (Susanna). The boys were horrified. Esther pointed out that John was the groom after all, but that wouldn't mollify them. "He's a boy, and it's playing dress up. You can't do that—you're trying to feminize him!"

Gender Distinctions

When parents ignore God-created gender distinctions and roles, the entire human race suffers, especially little children. Contraception, abortion, infanticide, homosexuality, and other forms of child neglect and abuse are so often the fruits of ignoring God-created gender distinctions, roles, and responsibilities. Adults become obsessed with their own needs, pleasures, and aspirations. They cannot take their eyes off themselves long enough to "give their child a chance." We would echo Dr. Denmark's observation that "children are the sorriest, most neglected creatures on earth these days."

It is not the aim of this chapter to fully explore the implications of those God-given distinctions; there are many other books available which challenge the reader on this subject. Nevertheless, I would encourage my readers to recognize the obvious: Men and women are created differently. What are the implications of this fact and how does it play out in parenting? Again, look to the Scriptures for your guide and do not ignore the wisdom of older, sometimes wiser generations.

One day my father came home with two tickets to an evening tent show in town. He did not ask my mother to go with him, because women in those days (especially those with young children) would never have thought of leaving home at night. So, I went with Papa because I was only ten and not old enough to be disgraced by going with my father to a performance of that type.

After a very dramatic program called "Ten nights in a Bar Room" [decrying enslavement to alcohol] the stage was cleared, lanterns were turned up, and out came a tall, pompous lady dressed in a black silk voile skirt over a taffeta petticoat. She wore a white blouse with a high collar, a watch on one shoulder, and glasses on another. She really looked important, a woman making a speech in that tent full of men!

The woman was speaking in favor of suffrage. She insisted that if women could vote, they would clean up politics, stop drunkenness, and stop young boys from smoking "coffin tacks." Voting privileges for women, so she claimed, would make a better world for children. I am sure that suffragette was just as sincere as any reformer that ever lived.

I remember being very impressed by the speaker. Woman suffrage sounded like a good idea to me. As a child, I assumed most women were wonderful like my mother. Surely women like my mother would change the world if given a chance.

In those days, most men did respect women. They tipped their hats to a woman, helped her in and out of a carriage, opened and closed doors for her, and rose to their feet if she entered a room. They would not smoke, tell off-color stories, or use bad language in her presence. Most women were not in the work place, but they were queens in their homes—queens in their so-called slavery and they ran the country without realizing it.[29]

Now, women are voting and in the workplace. They are competing with men in every sphere of society. In fact, "emancipated" women are drinking, smoking, and cursing, just like, or better than the men.

The tent show and the suffragette talk was more than a century ago. I wonder what that suffragette would say if she saw what our world was like 60 years [now 94 years] after women won the right to vote? What would she think if she were a pediatrician today and saw all the neglected children that I have seen?...Has our emancipation brought man up to a higher level of right living and better health, or has woman lowered her standards and lost all she was fighting for? Have women used this great blessing of "freedom" to give little children a better chance for health and happiness, or have we killed the goose that laid the golden egg?

Boundaries

A child needs boundaries in his play area and in his behavior. Just as a fence in the back yard provides physical safety, so behavioral boundaries bring emotional security. Children are confused and frustrated when allowed to do one thing one day and disallowed the next. It is up to the parents (with God's guidance) to establish limits and enforce them consistently. Expectations should be spelled out as well as the penalties for violating a rule.

Do you want your child to pick up his clothes after bathing? He must be required to do so until the habit is firmly established. If he doesn't follow through, reasonable penalties are necessary. Do you want him to speak respectfully to adults? Teach him specifically what that means and insist that he comply.

Anything you start with little people you have to keep up. Perform an action three times, and they will expect it to be repeated. "Consistency" should be written on every wall of your home.

During the latter part of the ninth century AD, pirates posed a terrifying threat to English coastal villages. At any moment, cruel Vikings or Saracen pirates could descend upon a poor, unprotected village, murdering, pillaging, and destroying.[30] Some of the pirates would wait until nightfall, creep stealthily up to homes, and steal children away while their parents were sleeping—what an analogy! These children were then sold as slaves, and lived lives of bondage, never to return to their beloved homes. The threat of pirates and loss of beloved children motivated fathers to bond together and build castles and village walls to protect their families.[31]

I have compared those village walls to the family policies we have erected in our home. Ultimately, only God can protect our children, but He most often uses parents and the boundaries they set up, to do so. As children grow, these boundaries take the form of family policies such as curfews, dress codes, entertainment standards, driving privileges, etc. We distinguish our family policies from the moral laws of Scripture.[32] Moral laws are non-negotiable; family policies may vary from household to household. However, wise parents will base their policies on the wisdom of biblical standards.

The following are some Bowman "boundaries." I am unveiling them to encourage my readers to establish their own.

Policy:

All family members participate in family devotions.

Purpose:

To develop knowledge of Scripture and love for Christ

Foundational Commandments:

First and Second Commandments

Policy:

Euphemisms for profanity ("gosh," "gee," etc.), and Scripture jokes are prohibited.

Purpose:

To encourage respect for God and His Word

Foundational Commandment:

Third Commandment

Policy:

Email privileges begin at age 14 with time limitations.

Purpose:

To discourage sloth and gossip and encourage good work habits

Foundational Commandment:

Fourth and Ninth Commandments

Policy:

Driving privileges begin at age 18. (Only then do our children receive a basic cell phone with no internet access.)

Purpose:

To preserve the safety of person and property

Foundational Commandments:

Sixth and Eighth Commandments

Policy:

Daughters are not allowed to travel in a car alone with any man unless we are very confident of his character, know his family well, and there is no particular mutual attraction.

Purpose:

Ensure safety and guard purity

Foundational Commandments:

Sixth and Seventh Commandments

Be careful in setting family policies. Do not look to parenting magazines or prevailing norms for guidance. Rather, pray for help, look to God's Word, be thoughtful, and consult others who have been successful in rearing children. Setting up policies can be especially difficult because moms and dads today are grappling with uncharted territory. Our parents did not contend with the challenges of Internet, video games, cell phones, rampant pornography, and the like. Parents must not allow themselves to be naive or overly indulgent. (Most modern parents fit this description.) Neither should they establish boundaries which are so restrictive that there is no room for children to grow. A healthy balance must be maintained.

When children are young, they should comply with our policies without discussion. As they grow, it is important that they learn the purpose behind family policies and the reasons why we expect certain behaviors. The boundaries are there to protect them until they have the wisdom and maturity to maintain personal codes of behavior.

Many parents wrongly assume that when a child turns 18, they automatically reach the age of "no accountability." Cultural norms encourage parents to release their eighteen-year-old children to complete social and moral independence, and from any familial responsibilities. In truth, becoming a legal adult does not release a young adult from a God-given obligation to the fifth commandment.[33]

Certainly, your relationship changes. As children grow older, gradually your role in their lives changes. Once you were a queen; now you are a coach. This doesn't mean that all family rules go out the window, but it does mean that young adults need room to make some decisions, mistakes, and transition into full adulthood. Ushering children into adulthood requires great care and constant prayer.

Adolescence can be the most miserable period of one's life. Bodily changes occur so fast it's difficult to keep up with them, and an adolescent struggles with identity—he's neither child nor adult. At that age, parents must change their approach, but not their standards of right and wrong. If children see a parent break down his or her standards, they lose respect for the parent.

"Don't do or say anything you'll regret later," I tell young people. "Once you've done or said something, you can never take it back. God can forgive, but you can't forget."

I encourage a young person to put a little note on his mirror which says something like this: "As long as I live in my parents' home, sleep in their bed, and eat their food, I will obey their rules. Someday I'll have a son or daughter of my own, and I will want him to obey my rules."

TLC

Mothering is an art requiring great sensitivity, perseverance, and wisdom. There are many balances to maintain as a mom nurtures her child. Family life and routine shouldn't revolve around a child's desires, or he will grow to be a tyrant and seldom content. He may never fully adjust to the reality that he isn't the center of the universe. There are many simple ways to build personal security without raising a tyrant.

Take the following inventory: Am I establishing eye contact with my child? Am I listening carefully to his words? Do I take time to answer questions thoughtfully (not necessarily every question)? Do I examine his handiwork seriously? Do I share in the joy of his accomplishments and sympathize with his sorrows? Do I praise him when he is good? Am I quick to give physical affection and encouragement?

Stop occasionally and do something that's fun with your child, even if it's very simple. I think with fondness of the time my grandmother mended my dress and sewed on a button for me. Together we searched through her button tin for one that matched. She let me choose. We took our time, and she even let me thread the needle—wow! I remember those beautiful buttons, my grandmother's smile and gentle hands! But, I especially cherish how comfortable and loved I felt sitting close beside Mama Lois while she listened to my prattle and sewed for me.

Dr. Denmark was a great example of one who gave TLC even in the midst of her busy schedule. On winter days she usually had a space heater in her office. After examining my children, she warmed their clothes in front of it before I redressed them. This simple but thoughtful act made little ones feel special.

My great-great-grandfather emphasized how vital it was to foster a confiding relationship with your child. This kind of relationship is simplest to gain when children are young and openhearted, before unnatural barriers of reserve have developed.

"How easy it is in early childhood to gain the intimacy and confidence to which I have referred. The little child naturally seeks to confide everything to its parent. Let but the slightest encouragement be given; let the little one only feel that there is a loving heart ready to sympathize with it; to rejoice with it; to solve patiently its difficulties; to bear forgivingly with its wrongs, and to lead it kindly by the hand through all the perplexities of its path; and how naturally, how unreservedly does it cast itself upon the bosom that seeks its confidence, and pour out there the very deepest and most sacred thoughts and feelings of its heart.

"And who shall say what advantage such a parent will have in the training of his child! He is like the physician who has had the full diagnosis of the disease he is to treat. He is like the lawyer to whom the client has fully unburdened his case. He knows how to direct the mind and mould the character of his child; and at the same time, as the result of this loving intimacy, he acquires an influence over it—the influence of mind over mind, and of heart over heart—the blessed results of which it is impossible to estimate.[34]

"Some of you have those about your knees who are still in tender childhood, whose hearts yearn for intimate communion with you. Take them home to your bosoms, in loving and confidential communication. Speak to them freely. Encourage them to keep back nothing from you. Let them see that you are worthy of their confidence; that you appreciate it; that you will cherish it as a sacred thing and keep it inviolate. Let your bosom be the willing receptacle of all that is joyous or sad, in their daily experience. Above all, let religion be the subject of frequent and intimate conversation. In your daily walks; by the evening fireside; and in the bed chamber, as the little form is composing itself for sleep, let words of tenderest religious counsel be imparted; inquiries after religious truth be awakened and answered; let your child feel and know all the deep, yearning anxieties of your soul for its early conversion to God. Do this, and the Holy Spirit will bless, as He has so often blessed with words of tender, confidential admonition to the awakening of a new life in the soul of your child; and while the endearments of the domestic circle will be enhanced a thousand fold by the loving confidence which such communion will beget, you may be the honoured instrument, in the hands of God, of conveying that living Word, by which the soul of your child shall be forever saved."[35]

Our streets and jails are full of people who have grown up without parental guidance. I've worked in the slums since 1928, and so many of them say the same thing: 'When I was a child, my parents didn't help me, didn't feed me. They had plenty of money but no time for me.'

Note: Avoid **excessive** praise and **excessive** familiarity with your children. A child should not be complimented so often that he presumes upon it and assumes he deserves praise every time he does right. If he is constantly commended but not required to obey or submit to the authorities in his life, that youngster is likely to become vain, prideful, impertinent, and insecure.

Nor should a parent become so familiar with his child that parental authority is undermined. In our super egalitarian society, parents tend to treat their children like little adults or buddies. It is assumed that this kind of relationship will foster mutual respect and greater maturity in children. Instead, excessive familiarity breeds indifference to parents' wishes and commands, and often cocky, overconfident attitudes.

It is important for parents to be humble and admit when they are wrong. However, that humility should not be expressed in a way that fosters contempt for a parent's wisdom or position. The parental transition from queen to coach must come gradually as the child grows and exhibits maturity, cooperation, and respect for authority. Teaching children to use titles is still a good idea (Mr., Mrs., ma'am, sir, etc.). Titles are good reminders of age distinctions and the need to respect authority.

Dreams

Children need to dream, to have something to yearn for. They love birthday parties and special events. Half the joy is in the anticipation. If birthday parties came every day, they would soon be old hat. Don't fulfill your children's wants instantly. Give them something to work for. Teach them to wait and anticipate.

Your daughter wants a new dress? Help her sew one. Your son wants a toy car? Tell him he might get it for Christmas. Maybe if he does some extra chores around the house, he can earn enough to purchase it himself.

Encourage your children to look forward to the future. What would they like to accomplish with their lives? What would they like to save their pennies for? Help them take the first steps toward fulfilling those goals.

It's depressing to look around and observe moral and economic decline in our culture. There's reason for discouragement and even outrage, yet in our pessimism let's not rob our children of their hopes. Young adults with no hope or initiative often escape into a pleasure-centered life, immersing themselves in video fantasy worlds, addictions, or immorality. Teach your children to use their imaginations to birth new ideas for industry, service, or invention. Inspire them with the truth that a life lived according to God's principles can have a huge impact in this world.

The happiest children in the world are those who have something to wish for, something to give them a thrill. But if they instantly get everything they want, there's no thrill. Christmas was a great time for us because we received gifts that were special, things we normally didn't get except once a year. There was an orange, nuts, raisins, toys, a doll perhaps. It was a thrill, but now a child is bought a new toy with every trip to the store. Where is the excitement? It's kind of like…well, modern marriage. If a couple's been living together before the wedding, what's the point in a honeymoon?

When I was eight years old and went off to school for the first time, it was really exciting. Our parents gave me a pencil box and a little book satchel. I looked forward to school as a new adventure. Children nowadays have been in institutions since they were six weeks old…. Now, there's no incentive to make a toy; they just go to the store and buy it. They don't have to read a book—just turn on the TV. There are no thrills for little kids anymore.

Work

Recently I spent two hours trying to get gum out of my son's dress shirts so he could wear them to a conference (somehow gum mysteriously ended up in my dryer). Whew! Looking back over 34 plus years of parenting eleven children, there have been countless dishes washed, diapers changed, loads of laundry...the list goes on. Was it worth it? I can answer with a resounding "yes!"

Through the years I have been motivated by the knowledge that work done *"as for the Lord"*[36] is always purposeful. Now that we have seen our children grow, learn, and become the individuals they are, it is even easier to realize the importance of those efforts that have gone into rearing a family. I hope our children will carry with them that sense of purposeful labor, even when work seems menial or obscure.

We live in a pleasure-oriented society. Everyone lives for the weekend. Actually, too much play in a youngster's life can bring listlessness and discontentment. Even a young child will find satisfaction in working hard and a job well done.

Teach your children to work hard and be thorough in whatever task they perform, being sensitive to their capabilities. Chores are a great way to start the training. John's job was to clear the dishes. "Johnny, do a good job for Jesus. Carry the plates carefully. Make sure you wipe off all those crumbs—not onto the floor. Scoop them into the cloth. Hey, you did a great job. It really encourages me to have a clean table. Thank you!"

Help your children discover their particular talents and diligently develop those God-given gifts. No matter what occupation a young man secures, he can have the knowledge that he is never a failure whose work is committed to Christ.

Why was I not born in the slums? I had a grandmother who knew how to work. She was widowed with two little girls to rear on her own. Not only did she care for her daughters, but she tended a big garden, sold eggs, and wove cloth from cotton she grew. She managed to save fifty cents a week to buy land that had to be cleared by hand.

Eventually, my grandmother had four-hundred acres and a good home for my mother and aunt. She taught my mother that it was a sin not to work, and a sin not to give thanks for work; but to do every job as though she were working for the Giver of all things. I was saved the tragedies that have befallen so many children because of a grandmother and a mother who believed in God and work.[37]

Some children break their toys in a temper and mama will say, "Now don't cry; I will buy you another one." That child is not likely to ever take care of anything, for he has learned he can destroy and yet have—which is not true [in real life].... Destruction and extravagance are the forerunners of a great many heartaches a parent has to face. For a person to succeed he must learn the value of money, how it is made, and how it should be spent.[38]

Teamwork

A family should learn to function as a team. Scripture says: *"Two are better than one because they have a good return for their labor. For if either of them falls, the one will lift up his companion."* [39] A team does much better than one alone. If one of its members is ailing, others are there to pitch in.

Many of today's children view their parents as facilitators for their own desires. Mom and Dad exist to provide the money and transportation necessary to fulfill their wants. In contrast, let's train our children to see themselves as part of a cooperative effort, working toward accomplishing God-given family goals. They need to see their responsibility toward their family, not just to themselves. Teamwork means working together and taking turns.

Chores should be shared among all according to ability. Naturally, older members have the most responsibility, but no one should be unfairly burdened with work.

If sister is sick, other siblings ought to take up the slack and cheerfully help with her chores because their turn will come. Does brother have a special event coming up? Sister should be willing to baby-sit while mother takes him shopping for a new shirt. Instead of being jealous, everyone can be proud of him when he performs. Was baby born with a physical handicap? The whole family ought to view him as their corporate responsibility to encourage, give therapy, and help with his special challenge.

Numerous examples illustrate that kind of cooperation. The sooner parents inculcate the concept in their children, the better. Even two-year-old Joseph can help six-year-old Esther set the table by placing the napkins. The younger a child understands he's part of a team effort, the less likely he is to resent chores and responsibilities. "Many willing hands make light and joyous work!" It's a great old saying!

Note: Our family has enjoyed the blessing of older children conducting a home-based business. Money-making, young adults can pay younger siblings to cover their share of household chores. This arrangement makes everybody happy!

We must teach our children to keep the Sabbath, to take that day to rest the body and to get spiritual strength for the coming week. The second half of this commandment is just as important as the first half if a person is to be secure...it is just as sinful not to work six days as it is to work on the Sabbath. If this commandment were kept, there would be no want on earth [and nobody expecting free lunches].

> Children must be taught that everything we have, somebody had to work for and that nobody owes them a living... They cannot ride through life on a boat built by someone else, but they must make their own. Children must be taught that work is truly a gift of God and is something to be thankful for, not something to be feared.[40] Work should be seen as a privilege and a pleasure, not a punishment.

Ministry

Charity begins at home; ministry among family members. Daddy could use a back rub after a long day's work. Is little sister sick? Maybe making her a get-well card or reading her a story would be comforting. Mom looks tired; brother could offer to do some grocery shopping so she could take a break (I like this one).

Children learn to serve in the home, ministering to "neighbors" who are closest. That servant-hearted attitude should also extend to those outside the home, particularly within our church community as well as others less fortunate than we, who may need us. We all have a natural tendency to become self-centered and feed that self-centeredness in our children by focusing exclusively on their needs and desires.

Dr. Denmark's former patients may remember a wooden sign posted on her clinic door announcing her weekly hours of practice. On Thursdays the clinic was closed, and not because it was Dr. Denmark's day off. Every Thursday, she volunteered her time at Central Presbyterian Clinic until it closed. For 56 years, she treated thousands of little children whose parents could not afford any medical care.

Involve your children, especially the older ones, in serving others. Most church communities provide plenty of opportunity— collecting clothes for a crisis pregnancy outreach, baby-sitting for a sidewalk counselor, visiting a neglected senior citizen, helping cook a meal or cleaning for a new mother, using their pennies to sponsor a child overseas, working in a soup kitchen, or just being a good listener and friend to a lonely person.

Children can help fill some very real needs, and it's excellent for their growth in character to be involved this way. A few words of caution are needed: As you minister to others outside your family, remember the priority of protecting your children from harmful influences. Also, when children are young, outside ministry usually means extra time on the road for mom. As important as ministries are, be realistic in evaluating the time required for them. Don't become so overburdened that essential household chores are neglected. Your ministry to your home is vital and mustn't be sacrificed for any extended period of time. Maybe Daddy or big brother can help with the chauffeuring!

I had a preacher's wife in my office one day. Her baby looked like the wrath of God. She said, "I want you to understand one thing, Dr. Denmark. My husband is a minister. I'm called to do so many things; I don't have time for this baby."

"Maybe you'd better go upstairs and read my Bible," I said. "It doesn't read like that. Mine says, 'Start in Jerusalem and go to Judea.'" If you bear a child, there's no sacrifice too great for that baby.

Like Dr. Denmark, I was blessed to have hardworking parents and grandparents. I have never known two more resilient, energetic, and servant-hearted people than Hugh and Betty Linton, my parents. They poured their lives out in service on the mission field. Both were well-educated and cultured people, but never shrank from performing the most menial tasks associated with church planting and caring for those with tuberculosis, leprosy, mental disorders, and other illnesses.

Dad was a minister, but his huge hands were always calloused and stained from manual labor, and his invigorating spirit never failed to brighten a room. Mom, at 87, is still serving. In 2010, her beautiful home burnt to the ground while she was on a "mission trip." All carefully archived family records, artifacts, antiques, and treasures were destroyed. Her few surviving possessions after the fire were mostly in her suitcase. We were afraid for her mental health.

"You don't have to worry about me," she reassured us. "Don't you know I believe the things I've told you—our true treasures are in heaven…but I'm going to rebuild. The grandchildren enjoyed my house so much. They need a place to gather and create memories."

I hope that I can follow the example my parents set for me in serving the people God has placed in my life.

Adversity

The first time our baby, Malinda, bloodied herself was on the edge of a coffee table. She was just learning to stand. I still remember the silky little head bobbing up and down as she pulled to a standing position. There was a goofy, elated smile of triumph and then—whoops—a slip and the poor little chin connected with unyielding wood. The sweet smile suddenly disappeared and wailing began. I was probably more distressed than she was—bad coffee table!

A mother's first instinct is to shield her child from hurt, and to comfort, console, and protect. These instincts are absolutely essential to the well-being of children. However, life is full of disappointments, pain, and troubles; and parents cannot completely shield their children. Also, it is through bumps and bruises that a toddler masters walking and children learn caution. We mature through hard times. The wise parent shields her child from harm, but also trains him to grow through adversity and face it with courage.

"Adversity training" begins early: Susanna was terribly disappointed—the flu and fevers hit on Christmas Eve. John, the board game whiz, lost at chess three times in a row. Leila was so looking forward to the picnic, and it rained all weekend. Christina's new kitten disappeared. Emily's carefully tended squash plant withered. In the scheme of life, these are minor troubles, but they loom larger in the mind of a child and provide great opportunities for adversity training.

A child who is easily discouraged or filled with self pity and bitterness when things go wrong needs encouragement, but also firm admonishment. If he learns cheerful resignation when minor trouble ensues, he will be much more prepared to handle true tragedy when it arrives. If he perseveres through minor obstacles, he will more likely be strong when major obstacles appear on the scene.

The parent who has learned to handle adversity himself, by believing and acting on the promises in God's Word, is the best teacher for his child in these circumstances. He can demonstrate proper responses through his own example and by "practically teaching and applying principles at the level of the child's ability to comprehend."[41]

True children of God can possess deep confidence that adversity (small or great) comes from the hand of a merciful, sovereign Father who can be trusted with our present and future. Whatever adversity we face has purpose. He can be trusted with our happiness. Actually, true happiness is not a product of ideal circumstances but "a by-product of a life lived daily in diligent pursuit of righteousness and the glory of God."[42]

Nurture patience, trust, prayerfulness, determination, strength, courage, and gratitude in the garden of your child's heart. Pull the weeds of bitterness, self-pity, resentment, jealousy, anxiety, and an easily defeated spirit.

Note: Here is a good quote reflective of Proverbs 24:16. "Success is not final. Failure is not fatal. The courage to keep trying is what counts."[43]

We must let the child make some mistakes and see them fail. I remember how my child at four years decided to get rich quick. She fixed up a box on the front lawn, had our wonderful old cook make her a big pitcher of lemonade, got some cups out, took a chair, and sat in the hot sun waiting for someone to come along and buy, but nobody came. I kept watching and hoping someone would come and buy just one cup, but no one did. I felt the urge to go out and buy it all myself. She stayed out there a long time, then gathered up her equipment and came in. I did not say a word, for I knew she had many disappointments ahead of her and this was a good lesson to teach her how to meet the big ones to come... It is hard to sit by and see a child disappointed, but the earlier children learn they can't have everything they think they want, the better it is. These lessons can be taught best by the child's parents.[44]

Hardships don't all come at one time; they are like the storms against an oak tree. Each storm makes the tree send down stronger roots. One might say the tree was foolish to start out knowing it would be hit by storms thousands of times, but the little tree, like the teenager, takes the days as they come and grows with the hardships. We parents must see this in our teenagers and advise rather than command. We must give them a true picture of what we felt and did at their age, how our lives have been, the pitfalls we encountered, and how we solved our problems. They must be talked to like adults and must learn how mature adults talk and act.

> We must show [our young adults] they must look to something greater than parents to hold them up. They must bring their problems to a God that gives life and strength to all who will use and develop the life they have in keeping with their talents and capabilities.[45]

I spent many hours in conversation with Dr. Denmark through the years. Not once did I detect in her the slightest taint of bitterness or personal grievance. She always maintained an air of gratitude to God and others. Having lived over a century, Dr. Denmark undoubtedly experienced many heartaches, trials, disappointments, and physical discomforts.

In my last lengthy conversation with her, she expressed gratitude for her family, husband, and even the mothers of her patients. "I would not have been able to help any children had their mothers not been willing to follow through with my instructions. I could have said all the right things, but somebody had to be willing to go home and do the right things. I have been blessed all these years in the wonderful mothers who brought their children to me."

Christ

The focus of this book is clearly family health issues. Yet physical health can never be fully separated from one's spiritual condition before the Creator of our bodies. Health habits, time priorities, and family relations are all critically important, but pale in significance next to our need for spiritual cleansing before a wonderful and holy God.[46]

Sickness, pain, and death are not normal entities; they became commonplace intruders when true moral guilt and spiritual death shattered the tranquility of Eden.[47] Apart from moral cleansing and spiritual rebirth, there is no hope of true life or complete healing, but certain expectation of eternal misery and death. Contrary to what many wish and philosophize, there are not many paths to God. There is only one path which leads to true salvation. That path is a Person.[48]

The Scripture tells us about a time when Jewish mothers brought their children to Jesus to be blessed.[49] His disciples rebuked them, probably thinking He was too busy with other more consequential matters than to be bothered with children. But Jesus was indignant and intervened; He was never too busy for little ones. Jesus took them in His arms, blessed them and said, *"The kingdom of God belongs to such as these."*[50] What a tender, remarkable story. What a consolation to those mothers.

Are we willing to follow their example in bringing our children to Christ? Do we pray for them and show them the Person of Christ as He is presented in the Bible? What about taking them to a Bible-believing church to gain true knowledge of the Savior?

Children need to understand life as God intended it to be, learning to see it through the "spectacles" of Scripture. They need to repent of their sins and learn how to live by the Ten Commandments. Teach them to study the Bible, to solve problems and find answers according to the principles found in God's Word.

As soon as our little ones learn to read, they are encouraged to read the Bible upon rising each morning. Our family also studies, discusses, and memorizes Scripture together after breakfast while everyone is still seated at the table. Scripture memory is followed by prayer with each family member taking turns. After supper we read a good Bible story book, sometimes sing a hymn, and close with prayer again. This simple routine keeps us consistent. Some of my favorite Bible study aids are: *The Child's Story Bible* by Catherine F. Vos, *Leading Little Ones to God* by Marian M. Schoolland, *Balancing the Sword* by Alan B. Wolf, and *Matthew Henry's Commentary*. *The Child's Catechism* (for younger children) and *The Shorter Catechism* (for older children) are wonderful summaries of the teachings of the Bible. We study and memorize the question and answers.

The essence of mothering is to discern the true needs of our offspring and give of ourselves sacrificially to meet them. The wisest parent maintains her own health—physical and spiritual—and comes to God for guidance. Surely the One who made your children knows what is most essential for them.

Come to Jesus and bring your children to Him. At His feet, you will discover life. You and yours will learn what is truly needful... as Mary of Bethany did long ago.

Notes

1. Luke 10:41b-42
2. Matthew 6:33
3. Charles Hummel, *Tyranny of the Urgent* (Downers Grove, IL: InterVarsity Press, 1967)
4. Ephesians 6:1-3
5. Reverend Jerry White, "Training Children in Preparation for Godliness" Proverbs 22:6, Bold Ministries
6. Leila Daughtry-Denmark, M.D., *Every Child Should Have a Chance* (Atlanta, GA: 1971), 152
7. Denmark, *Every Child Should Have a Chance*, 100, 151
8. Matthew 20:20-28
9. Denmark, *Every Child Should Have a Chance,*126-127
10. Ephesians 5:22-32
11. Philippians 4:19
12. Denmark, *Every Child Should Have a Chance*, xiv, 162-163
13. Denmark, *Every Child Should Have a Chance*, 66
14. Hummel, *Tyranny of the Urgent*
15. Jacob Abbott, *Training Children in Godliness*, ed. Michael J. McHugh (Arlington Heights, IL: Christian Library Press, 1992), 114–16
16. Harvey Newcomb, *How to Be a Lady* (Boston, MA: Gould, Kendall, and Lincoln, 1850), 173
17. 1 Timothy 5:13; II Thessalonians 3:11-12

18. Hebrews 10:24
19. Denmark, *Every Child Should Have a Chance*, 174
20. Denmark, *Every Child Should Have a Chance*, 174
21. Reverend T.D. Witherspoon, D. D., *Children of the Covenant* (Richmond, VA: Presbyterian Committee of Publication, 1873), 208
22. Witherspoon, *Children of the Covenant*, 209
23. Witherspoon, *Children of the Covenant*, 210
24. Witherspoon, *Children of the Covenant*, 211
25. Witherspoon, *Children of the Covenant*, 212-213
26. Denmark, *Every Child Should Have a Chance*, 84
27. Denmark, *Every Child Should Have a Chance*, 88
28. Denmark, *Every Child Should Have a Chance*, 90
29. Denmark, *Every Child Should Have a Chance*, 207
30. Joseph and Francis Gies, *Life in a Medieval Castle* (New York, NY: Harper and Row, 1974), 12
31. Geoffrey Botkin, *Father to Son* (The Western Conservatory of the Arts and Sciences DVD, 2008)
32. Exodus 20
33. Exodus 20:12
34. Witherspoon, *Children of the Covenant*, 200-201
35. Witherspoon, *Children of the Covenant*, 205-206
36. Colossians 3:23
37. Denmark, *Every Child Should Have a Chance*, 147
38. Denmark, *Every Child Should Have a Chance*, 196-197
39. Ecclesiastes 4:9–10
40. Denmark, *Every Child Should Have a Chance*, 171
41. Reverend Jerry White
42. Reverend Jerry White
43. Reverend Jerry White
44. Denmark, *Every Child Should Have a Chance*, 103-104
45. Denmark, *Every Child Should Have a Chance*, 126
46. Psalm 51, Matthew 15:1-20, Mark 7:1-23, Luke 5:17-26, Hebrews 9
47. Genesis 2:17, Genesis 3
48. Acts 4:12
49. Mark 10:13–16; Matthew 19:13–15; Luke 18:15–17
50. Mark 10:14

Recommended Parenting Resources

The following is a list of resources I have found helpful in training my children. With any human resource (including this book) the reader is advised to exercise discernment. Not every bit of counsel should be accepted at face value. Instead, a parent should prayerfully read and listen, all the while asking the question, "Does this comply with Scriptural principles?"

The Holy Bible, particularly the book of Proverbs

Every Child Should Have a Chance, by Dr. Leila Denmark

Well-Fed, Well-Rested Baby (DVD), Windy Echols and
    Tammy Seagraves

The Duties of Parents, by John Charles Ryle

Under Loving Command, by Pat Fabrizio

Raising Godly Children in an Ungodly World
    DVD series),by Michael and Susan Bradrick

Hints on Child Training, H. Clay Trumbull

Child Training Tips, by Reb Bradley

To Train Up a Child, by Michael and Debi Pearl

Withhold Not Correction, by Ray Bruce

What the Bible Says About Child Training, by Richard Fugate

Shepherding a Child's Heart, by Ted Tripp

Growing Kids God's Way (18 lesson lecture series), by Gary Ezzo

Institute in Basic Youth Conflicts
    (hard-bound workbook with course), by Bill Gothard

The Shaping of a Christian Family, by Elizabeth Elliot

The Family, by J.R. Miller

The Family, by B.M. Palmer

What is a Family?, by Edith Schaeffer

❧ 13 ☙
Vaccinations

One of Dr. Leila Denmark's greatest accomplishments was her work over an 11-year period on the vaccine for pertussis. She received the 1935 Fisher Award for outstanding research in diagnosis, treatment, and immunization of whooping cough.

In light of modern controversy over routine vaccinations, the following interview with Dr. Denmark is especially relevant. Her perspective on how they should be administered was based on extensive experience beginning with that research and extending through her years of practice. Because of the longevity of her practice, she probably vaccinated more children than any one physician in the world today.

(This particular interview was conducted by the author during the early nineties. The exact date was not recorded.)

Q. "Dr. Denmark, one of the greatest accomplishments of your life has been the vital part you played in developing the pertussis vaccine. I understand it's the same one given routinely to infants in DPT shots (the P in DPT standing for pertussis). Will you trace for us the history of how you developed it and what prompted your work?"

A. "In 1932 I saw about three lines in the *Journal of the American Medical Association* saying that some doctor was speculating about a possible vaccine for whooping cough. His name was Sauer. At that time, I had an enormous group of kids sick with it at Central Presbyterian Church Baby Clinic. I had lost triplets at Grady Hospital. I had twins with inter cranial hemorrhages, and a world of patients losing all their meals and having seizures every four hours. Something had to be done. At that time I heard of a man in East Point who had it and had fractured two ribs and hemorrhaged in his eyes from coughing. I went to his house and asked if he would let me have some of his blood (I wouldn't do that today because that would be "terrible"). I took 100 cc. and put it in the icebox. The next morning I took the serum off and injected a child subcutaneously with it. It cured him like magic. Then I knew there was something we could do.

"One of the most interesting things I discovered at that time was that I could use a mother's blood to cure her sick baby if she had had whooping cough herself. If a nursing baby had been sick for about a week, I took 100 cc. of his mother's blood, took the serum off, and put it in subcutaneously. The antibody response was just as good as when I used the East Point man's blood. Of course that, too, was terrible. Today we're afraid of AIDS. I'd be put in jail. But I proved my point...there was something we could do to help these children.

"Understand, if a patient has suffered whooping cough for the full six weeks, the disease runs its course, and he is immune for life. However, if the disease is cured through antibiotics or serum, the patient doesn't develop permanent immunity because he hasn't built up enough antibodies. I realized we needed an effective vaccine, so I wrote Eli Lilly Company to ask them if they would make one I could test... like Dr. Sauer's. I did hundreds of vaccinations with it and all kinds of blood tests to determine the level of immunity that developed. I ended up using a complement fixation test to determine immunity. I gave those kids the vaccine that Lilly sent me. About 25 percent of them showed a 4+ on the complement fixation. It wasn't enough, so I asked Lilly to double the strength. I found we did far better with that. Two more times I asked them to double it again and found that 99 percent of those children got the same antibody response they would have from a full case of the disease. They were immune. But I didn't do the research all by myself—Eli Lilly, Cutter, Emory Public Health Department, and a lot of other people helped.

"For many years I continued taking serum from my vaccinated children and sending it to the two drug companies to test for immunity. Then I found a very interesting procedure called an agglutination test. I took a drop of blood from a child's finger and put it with the antigen. In a minute I could determine whether the vaccinations had effectively immunized the child."

Q. "Didn't you use this same test up until a few years ago? I believe you tested my oldest daughter after her DPTs."

A. "That's right. But Lilly quit making the vaccine, and I couldn't get the antigen. Cutter made me some, but it didn't work. So a few years ago, I quit testing my patients for an antibody response."

Q. "Did you do research on when the vaccine should be administered?"

A. "Yes, and I found out something that was critical. I began by vaccinating a pregnant mother, thinking I could immunize the baby inside her. The antibody response was no good. After birth, when the baby was a month old, I gave him a shot, but it didn't work; at two months it didn't work, and so on. I began to get a wonderful response about the fifth month. I discovered that until then the child's immune system isn't mature enough to respond effectively."

Q. "Some now say the pertussis vaccine can cause dangerous reactions like encephalitis, seizures, convulsions, fever up to 106°, and breathing problems. They even accuse it of causing Sudden Infant Death Syndrome (SIDS or crib death). How do you feel about such allegations?"

A. "They're big lies! I've been using it since 1932 without ever encountering a severe reaction from it. I wouldn't pay any attention to such propaganda. There is always somebody tearing down things we try to do."

Q. "So you think the DPT vaccine is as good now as it was years ago?"

A. "That's right, but if it's given too early, it doesn't do any good. Sometimes they give it to sick kids and then blame the vaccine for the illness. I always give it in the deltoid muscle, not in the fat of the leg.

"I remember doing research down at McDonough, Georgia. A child had had the shots and was rumored to be paralyzed because of them. I had to investigate and asked the mother, 'How old was the baby when he held his head up?' He never had. 'How old was he when he turned over in bed?' He never had. They had been blaming his immobility on the vaccine, not realizing he had *amyotonia congentia*. There are so many cases like that. If they'd really study this thing, they would know there's nothing wrong with the vaccine.

"I could send a child to the hospital to get his tonsils out, and the next morning he might wake with a 106 degree temperature and break out with the measles. Some would say, 'Never take out tonsils because tonsillectomies cause measles.'

During a polio epidemic, a doctor in Cincinnati took a baby's tonsils out. The next morning the baby was paralyzed. Some said, 'Don't ever take tonsils out; the tonsillectomy paralyzed the child.' The child already had polio, but no one knew it. It's so easy to blame vaccinations for a concurrent condition. I wish people who say these things could just go back and see what it was like before. Vaccines are the greatest thing that ever happened for little children."

Q. "About Sudden Infant Death Syndrome. There is so much talk today about SIDS. Would you say a few words about it?"

A. "I've been practicing medicine for almost 70 years, and I've never had a SIDS baby, because I insist that mothers place their infants on their stomachs and instruct them how to make the baby's bed correctly (See pages 16-19).

"There are a lot of things that might make a baby die. A baby with meningitis can die in his sleep. But I don't believe an infant can get what we call SIDS unless he is placed on his back. I know I'm right. An infant on its back is in constant danger of asphyxiating on its own spit-up. The child may burp up a mouth full of milk and breathe it into his lungs, choking himself to death. It only takes a little thing to choke an infant to death.

"A man received a grant to study SIDS and did a lot of his research in countries where babies sleep on sheepskins. I can imagine one might smother if he was placed on his stomach with his face buried in thick wool. That particular researcher concluded an infant should always be placed on his back or side. Placing a baby on its back is potentially fatal. On his side he may not get SIDS, but he's unable to exercise his muscles properly and gets his little head out of shape. Babies need to use all four limbs and the muscles in their necks. They can't do that unless they are on their stomachs.

"I had a patient in here not long ago who was about four months old and had been put in one of those devices that kept him propped on his side. Four months old, and he couldn't hold his head up because he had never used the muscles in his neck! His right arm was weak and the side of his head was very flat.

"A baby placed on his stomach feels secure. He spits up onto the crib sheet without danger, can exercise his muscles well, and develops a nicely shaped head. It is so important."

Q. "What's the worst reaction a patient is likely to get from a DPT shot?"

A. "Four hours later there may be a little fever that lasts about 12 hours, but nothing more than that. Aspirin takes care of it. We used to give pertussis separately. It never caused a fever, but there was a little from the diphtheria and tetanus. So the temperature was from them, not the pertussis."

Q. "With actual whooping cough, you don't usually get fever."

A. "Not unless there is a secondary infection."

Q. "But with diphtheria and tetanus (the diseases), you do get fever."

A. "Oh, boy, you sure do!"

Q. "Have any of your fully inoculated patients ever contracted whooping cough?"

A. "Never. If you are vaccinated correctly, you'll never have it, and I don't believe you need more than those three DPT shots. Some of my former patients were vaccinated 62 years ago and never got it. My own daughter, Mary, is an example."

Q. "What if a child has only a single DPT?"

A. "It takes three DPT shots to be fully immunized. I believe I had used the vaccines separately for about 11 years, and then Dr. Kendrick put the DPT together. I did it about a week apart back then, but you could conceivably give them once a year until the series was completed. On the other hand, I believe you could give the shots once a day, and it wouldn't harm the patient. They are normally given a month apart."

Q. "Many people are concerned about giving a triple vaccination because the child's immune system is required to fight three toxins simultaneously rather than individually."

A. "Oh, that's ridiculous! Some say you can't eat proteins and starches in the same day. So you eat the meat one day and the vegetables the next. But the stomach has all kinds of enzymes and digestive juices to digest anything all the time. The body can incur three diseases at the same time and heal itself from them simultaneously, so we can also handle three vaccinations at once."

Q. "According to anti vaccine sources, the effects are potentially more severe than the disease itself. They claim the vaccines can be contaminated with animal viruses. Some point out that the chemical makeup of the vaccines is different and thereby potentially more dangerous than the actual disease. Certain researchers claim that injecting them directly into the body messes up the immune system and prevents it from responding effectively."

A. "I have just one answer to all that. From my many years of experience I find none of that is true."

Q. "Some researchers claim that diphtheria, pertussis, and tetanus were already on the decline before the

vaccinations were introduced, that the DPTs did not actually contribute to the decrease of these illnesses."

A. "Well, I think those researchers ought to go back to about 1932 or 1933 and see what things were like then. At that time, I had 75 cases of whooping cough at Central Presbyterian Clinic. We were having diphtheria, tetanus, and polio, too. None of those diseases were declining on their own, but now we have vaccines that stop them from happening."

Q. "How would you respond to those who insist that a significant percentage of cases were actually caused by the vaccines?"

A. "Oh, that's a farce."

Q. "If cases are now rare, why bother inoculating?"

A. "They're rare because most children, except some of the very poor, receive the vaccine. I had one family that didn't believe in it until the father happened to get whooping cough. He was terribly sick. Their five-month-old baby got it, too, and probably would have died without erythromycin. If you spoke to that daddy today, he would tell you whooping cough is still bad. He's become a convert who believes in the vaccine."

Q. "If people stopped getting it, the disease would increase again. Is this right?"

A. "We'd be right back to where we were, oh yes! We think we've completely eliminated smallpox because they've used the vaccine in all countries, so there's no more around. There hasn't even been any vaccine available for seven years. If someone came into the United States with smallpox, a lot of people would get it, but they wouldn't die the way they used to because we have antibiotics. People don't have to get secondary infections. For whooping cough, we've got chloromycetin or erythromycin. Both can cure it."

Q. "I've heard that there haven't been any recent cases of smallpox. Is that right?"

A. "Yes, and I don't think we're having any big measles now either."

Q. "But you're saying that there are enough cases of DPT that we need to keep vaccinating."

A. "Sure. The government has furnished vaccines for years, but there are a lot of poor people who have no way to go get it. Some people just don't bother. We still find the diseases, especially in the slums."

Q. "Do you think most mothers and perhaps doctors of my generation really understand the horror of such diseases?"

A. "Oh, no, I don't think so at all. They haven't seen little kids coughing for six weeks, having seizures every four hours, vomiting with each cough, unable to retain fluids. The horrible things they had to go through! They were choking to death, and you were beating their backs trying to get them to breathe again. A child with diphtheria can't breathe at all. You have to put a tube in his neck. A child with polio can't walk. They say war is hell, but I can't fully comprehend the horror of war because I've never been in one. If people had to experience these dreadful illnesses, they'd have an entirely different opinion."

Q. "Is there a difference between the effectiveness of the killed-virus polio vaccine and the live-virus (oral) version?"

A. "I don't see any."

Q. "What about the MMR (measles, mumps, and rubella) vaccination? Is it important?"

A. "Very! I know the measles part works, but I'm not so sure about the other two. I've had vaccinated patients who developed both, but not measles."

Q. "There are researchers who claim that incurring those childhood illnesses actually strengthens a child's immune system. Do you agree?"

A. "One does become immune by going through them, but they can impair one's health. The vaccine is just as strengthening to the immune system as having the disease, but there's no suffering. The diseases do lots of bad things to your body that vaccine doesn't—it's such a simple, easy way of avoiding illness."

Q. "What about flu shots?"

A. "I believe all flu is caused by H Influenza, a definite organism. In 1940, I had somebody make me a vaccine with H Influenza organisms, but I didn't use it as we do today. I started with a tenth of a cc and increased one-tenth each visit for 12 shots, but the kids still got the flu. I'm a hundred years old, and I suppose I've had it a hundred times. If you can't immunize by having a disease, there is no way you make an effective vaccine. You can't immunize against strep and staph, either."

Q. "Do you think that having it done each year can immunize you for that one particular year?"

A. "No, I don't think it does a thing. You can have flu three times in one winter. I don't think you can immunize against H influenza any more than you can against strep, or staph, or pneumcoccus which causes pneumonia."

Q. "What do you think of the newer vaccinations such as the HIb for spinal meningitis and hepatitis B now given to newborns in hospitals?"

A. "The HIb is similar to the influenza shot; I don't think it works. I used the flu shot for years, and it didn't seem to do any good. But I'm not going to criticize anybody's vaccine for the simple reason that when I was researching mine, I knew that I had to find a way to prove it. And these people have to test it. Now, I've never had a case of hepatitis in my practice. I don't believe the vaccine hurts, but I don't know whether it helps. That's the point."

"Immunizations and baby food are the greatest things that have ever happened on this earth for little people."

(For further information on immunizations see pages 43-45.)

❧ 14 ☙
Story Time

In the foyer of Dr. Denmark's office was a screen plastered with pictures of her patients. There must have been hundreds of smiling little faces representing only a fraction of the lives Dr. Denmark touched during her seventy-five years of practice. I loved looking at the photos: fat-cheeked cherubs, snaggle-toothed ballerinas; an Olan Mills Christmas shot with junior dressed in his red vest. If one looked closely enough, one could find a Bowman or two.

I often think each picture represents a story of the impact a faithful physician has on the life of a family. Each story is a tiny thread in a beautiful tapestry of one life spent serving others. I've heard many of them and want to share a few with you.

Generations

Dr. Denmark may never know how much she means to me and my family. Before I had a child, my husband's grandmother spoke of the wonderful doctor to whom she had taken her three children. My mother-in-law in turn had taken hers there. They both mentioned how she made managing children and home so natural, what a great person she is, and how just knowing her enriched their lives. Of course, it was Dr. Denmark.

When my own daughter was born it would have been only natural to do the same, but I wasn't quite smart enough to follow their advice immediately. I selected a doctor a little nearer home, thinking all pediatricians were alike. Virginia was a beautiful, healthy baby, and before she was born I had decided to nurse her. It worked pretty well at first, but she soon started fussing about an hour after feeding. The problem grew worse until she was crying constantly. The doctor diagnosed her with reflux and eventually prescribed Zantac to be given after feedings. When she was four months old we were to go on our first out-of-town trip. Totally exasperated with her crying all morning, I kept asking myself how I would be able to deal with it in a small car for three hours. Almost as an answered prayer, the thought came: take her to Dr. Denmark. I put my sweet, pitiful baby in the car and went directly to the miracle worker I had heard so much about. It was a busy day for the good doctor, so we had to wait a while. But my nerves calmed as we sat watching the happy, well-behaved children in her care. I just knew she would have an answer to my precious child's problem.

Dr. Denmark asked a few brief questions as she examined Virginia.

"Was she nursed or bottle fed?" I had stopped producing milk and was feeding her formula. "How much was she taking at a time?" I'd been told to give her six ounces of milk at a feeding. "What else is she getting?" They hadn't even mentioned other food yet. She looked at me and said, "This child is starving. She should be getting eight ounces of milk and protein, vegetables, fruit, and a starch." I was horrified. Here I lived amid abundance, and my innocent baby was starving! I was ashamed. I loved my child and wanted the very best for her, yet I wasn't even feeding her enough. Dr. Denmark smiled.

"I think we can save her," she said. She sat me down and gave me a list of what Virginia should eat. She also explained how to prepare her meals and maintain a common-sense schedule.

I went straight home, threw away the expensive medicine, and fed her as instructed. Then we left to see my parents for the weekend. Her proud grandparents were amazed at how well she ate. Her mood was better, and she went straight to sleep that night instead of crying until one or two o'clock in the morning.

At this writing Virginia is sixteen months old. I have taken her only to Dr. Denmark since that day. She is happy, goes to bed on schedule, and sleeps well. Everything my husband's grandmother and mother told me about raising a child under Dr. Denmark's care I have found to be absolutely true. People say that I am lucky to have such a wonderful daughter. Lucky? I don't think so. God sent us Virginia, but we are blessed to know Dr. Leila Daughtry Denmark and benefit from her vast knowledge and experience.

—Denise Garner Jacob
Alpharetta, Georgia

Dr. Denmark has always been an angel in my life. Not only has she cared for my children for fifteen years but was my own pediatrician too. When I first took the children to her, Brooke was five, and I had recently had twin daughters. I was disillusioned with the medical profession, having gone through five years of high bills accumulated from scores of visits, not to mention prescriptions. I've never been a believer in dosing my family with drugs for every ache or pain. I knew Brooke's surface problems must stem from a bigger root problem and wanted to find out what it was. That was when someone told me I should go to Dr. Denmark.

I was surprised to learn she was still active, but I packed a lunch and some picture books, and we went to see a friendly face from my past. "She's ageless!" I thought when I saw her. Could it be that she's wearing the same uniform? My thoughts were quickly redirected as she began to examine the children. The twins were put on her infamous "green mush": beans, cereal, vegetables, cooked fruit and bananas, pureed and fed three times a day; only water to drink; and absolutely nothing between meals.

Next it was Brooke's turn. It was deja vu as I saw my daughter climb onto the tall wooden examining table where I used to sit. As she began her examination, Dr. Denmark talked with Brooke in a sweet and personable way, her comments always carrying a positive word of encouragement.

"This is such a fine young lady. I don't think I'd sell her." Brooke and I watched and listened in awe. After a thorough going-over, from blood work to feeling the skin on her back and closely checking her hair, she looked at me and asked if anyone had ever told me Brooke was allergic to milk.

"No, never," I said as I thought of all the milk I poured into her daily.

"Let me tell you what you've been going through with this child," she said. As if actually experiencing it, she spoke of the ear infections, rounds of antibiotics, and head colds Brooke had suffered for the past five years.

"She probably has tubes in her ears," she added. Everything she named was right on course. Then she sat me down and began spelling it all out. With her hemoglobin at sixty, Brooke was anemic. "Most doctors won't tell you that isn't normal, but it's not. Everyone's hemoglobin should be at one hundred. You'll never be healthy if your hemoglobin is low. If you do what I say, we can get these children well. If you don't, then don't tell anyone I'm your doctor," she said. I can hear those words as if it were yesterday. No one had ever spoken to me in such a firm yet loving way. I knew she genuinely cared. She began explaining how the digestive system works, talking about her great dislike for milk and blaming it for the anemia among so many children.

"Not even animals go back on milk after they're weaned," she remarked. "But humans do. It takes at least two weeks to get milk out of one's system and that includes all dairy products." I should have been taking notes. I asked her if she wanted us to come back in two weeks.

"No," she said, "if you do what I say, you won't need to. And if not, then don't waste your time or mine." With that I knew she meant business. She indeed wanted to see my children happy and healthier, and I appreciated her candor. On the way home, I remembered how she used to tell my mother to feed us black-eyed peas and cabbage. Best food on earth. And boy, did Mother obey! I think we had black-eyed peas and cabbage at least once a week, forever. Mother didn't let us eat between meals either. Well, it worked for me, so it would work for my children. We were about to make some lifestyle changes. Brooke's skin cleared up as did her congestion. Basically the girls' health has improved to the point that about all they need now is a yearly check-up.

—Jan Holland
Marietta, Georgia

With Love

Dr. Denmark has been an incredible mentor, doctor, and friend to all of my family! My twins, Preston and Jack, appeared on NBC television with her back in 1989 when they were a year old.

She has helped so much with my daughter. When Natalie was an infant, my husband and I took her to see Dr. Denmark because of a feeding problem, though we had been on her schedule from day one. She told us she would like to watch Natalie eat. Shortly afterward, she threw up all over the floor. I hurried to hand her to Joe so I could clean up the mess. Well, Dr. Denmark wouldn't hear of it. She insisted on getting down on her hands and knees and doing it herself —at ninety years old! She insisted I sit with my sweet baby. She has told me many times, "There is no more beautiful picture in all the world than a happy baby with its mother. There is no more pure love in the world than that." Well, maybe not. I usually don't argue with Dr. Denmark, but the love she gives to all her patients and their families comes mighty close!

—Liz May
Watkinsville, Georgia

Dr. Denmark is a remarkable woman. I began going to her when my daughter was three. Mollie had a chronic ear infection and was scheduled to have tubes put into her ears. My husband and I were uncomfortable at the idea and decided to try Dr. Denmark as a last resort.

"She has the kind of ears they like to put tubes in; don't let them! We'll give her antibiotics round the clock for seventy-two hours, and she'll be well," she said after one look. She didn't know why we were there—she just discovered the problem during a general exam. Mollie never had a recurrence!

Not only is Dr. Denmark the finest pediatrician I know, but she has shown us the kind of love and devotion that's hard to find. In January, 1994, I called her in a panic because seven-month-old R.J. was constipated and in extreme pain. She told me to immediately go to the children's emergency room. In very serious condition, my son was diagnosed with Hirschbrung's disease and treated. They suggested surgery be considered to correct it, but we should try medical maintenance for a few months first. R.J. did fine for about six weeks, then started having problems because his immune system was weakened. Three times in one month I had to call Dr. Denmark on her day off. All three times she had us come in and meet her at the office. When I told her the first time what had happened, her reply astonished me.

"I am so relieved to see him," she said. "For weeks I've been wondering about and praying for a child with this condition, whoever it was." She really believed R.J. would overcome the disease if we stuck with the program he was on. So far, it's working well.

I truly believe God put Dr. Denmark on earth to not only heal children and educate parents but also to encourage mothers in their line of duty. She has lifted me up and made me feel that what I am doing is the greatest "job" I could ever have. How right she is.

—Nancy Eldredge
Lithia Springs, Georgia

Reprieve

At three months, my John Matthew had colic so badly he got no sleep day or night. He screamed and threw up everything he'd ingested. Dr. Denmark put him on a variety of solid foods along with cooked oatmeal, and the food stayed down. He was a different baby! After seeing numerous pediatricians with no help except the hollow words, "He'll outgrow it," I was so relieved. I'll never forget her wise words and gentle nature.

—Nancy Pyle
Roswell, Georgia

It was back in 1988 that I first heard about Leila Denmark from a gas station attendant. He had asked if my two-week-old in the car seat beside me had been sleeping through the night. I looked at him, puzzled, wondering how anyone could ask such a crazy question. As a first-time mother I was beyond exhausted. Cameron had been getting me up countless times at night ever since I brought him home. I thought it was normal. How could a baby sleep through the night? Well, the attendant's nine kids had all done so after their third night home. He said Dr. Denmark had the solution.

"Where is this woman?" I asked. He gave me directions, and I went the very next day, taking a pregnant friend with me. We found the humble office with a sign on the door saying "Closed Thursdays." But I had to see her! Maybe I should come back the next day...but how could I survive another night! I saw a big white house next door that was probably hers. She must have seen the desperation on my face when I knocked on the door.

"Let's go have a look at your baby," she said. We walked over to her office, and God gave me two hours with that wise woman. How I wished for a tape recorder. Her words were full of such simple common sense. It seems we make life so complicated for ourselves, but Dr. Denmark speaks of what matters in life and how important these little lives are. She is remarkable.

"Put the baby to bed, making sure he's fed and changed and burped. Then make sure there isn't a snake in his crib and leave: meaning leave him alone. Let him cry; it's good for him." Wit and wisdom, what a mix.

"What can I do that's good for my pregnancy?" my friend asked.

"Laugh a lot," Dr. Denmark replied. For a two-hour consultation, the bill was eight dollars. After being with this special lady, you know she is one of God's gifts to our children.

—Leigh Smith Mintz
Roswell, Georgia

Before taking my first baby to Dr. Denmark I had been nursing her on demand and allowing her to sleep when she would. If she cried for more than five minutes, I picked her up to comfort her. By the time she was three months old, my nerves were shattered from lack of sleep, my husband was wondering if he would ever have a meal and clean clothes again, and I was feeling desperate.

Dr. Denmark had me put my daughter on a schedule, assuring me that it was not only all right to let her cry but that it was actually good for her. Crying helps clean out the nose and strengthens the lungs.

Within a week, we had a much happier home. The baby and I were both sleeping all night. My outlook improved. I was no longer "leaking" through the night. I was soon able to prepare good, balanced meals for us all using Dr. Denmark's schedule as a guideline. It was comforting to know that what I fed my family would be building healthier bodies. With my once-colicky baby contentedly in her playpen, Mommy was able to catch up on the housework.

—*Nora Dolberry Pitts*
Dallas, Georgia

Answers

I am the mother of three girls and three boys and met Dr. Denmark when my third child was ten months old. A friend of mine heard him wheezing one day and suggested I see Dr. Denmark.

At the time of my first visit in 1989, he was anemic and had ear and gastrointestinal infections. She said he probably had asthma that he would outgrow when he was five to nine years old, and that has held true for him. She told me to throw away the bottle and baby formula, start him on her diet, and give antibiotics every three hours for seventy-two hours (with the alarm clock set). I followed her directions, and he was soon better. He was also to avoid soy products. She told me to try a hot bath and give a baby aspirin for his wheezing attacks. It worked extremely well; we do it when any of the children have a bad cold. She suggested a dehumidifier in the basement, no carpet on his floor, no smoking in the house, and using bleach on any mildew in the house (i.e. bathroom, garage door, etc.). We still do all of those things today.

I kept my last three babies on her mashed food diet, and they have had no problems with food allergies or asthma. We also drink water—no juice, milk, or soda pop between meals. It has kept them from having any burning with urination.

We truly love Dr. Denmark. My children say it's like going to see a wonderful grandma. An office visit is a great spiritual experience. She takes the time to go over life, childrearing, and the wisdom of her many years with us.

—Celeste Frey
Cumming, Georgia

My first time meeting Dr. Denmark occurred when my daughter was nine months old. I was searching for a miracle for Dixie, a way out of putting tubes in her ears. The idea scared me; it seemed unnatural to put foreign objects in the body and expect them to be accepted. At four weeks Dixie went on a bottle because I dried up trying to breast feed a ten-pound baby. That's when the infections started—every two weeks we were in the doctor's office changing medicines because the last one didn't work. She got yeast infections from them. According to the dentist, violent throwing up and horrible fevers later on caused the enamel on her molars to crack.

The child had been through enough. It was time to find a doctor who would determine the cause, not just keep prescribing medicine after medicine. I learned of Dr. Denmark through my sister-in-law whose children had problems with rashes. On our very first visit she spent an hour with us and explained everything she was doing and why.

Gone were all dairy products, fruit juices, and sugar. If you had told me that just changing our way of eating would affect a child's ears, I would have said you were crazy. But it works; it really does! In three days we had a brand new Dixie, and she has never been bothered with ear infections again.

I pray the good Lord will send someone to study with her and pick up where she leaves off. Thanks, Dr. Denmark, you saved another child!

—Jannette Williams
Canton, Georgia

When All Else Fails

Dr. Denmark's a national treasure. Tom and I were blessed with twins on April 5, 1994. At the tender age of 42, I finally gave birth. Unfortunately the babies were eight weeks early. Thomas Justus weighed 4-1/2 pounds, while our Alexandra Justine weighed only 3-1/2 pounds. Alex had no medical problems except for her weight and stayed in the preemie nursery for a month. Thomas, however, had trouble.

A tiny valve in his heart didn't close completely. The theory is that it caused him to be without enough oxygen. The magnificent human body manages such a situation by robbing secondary organs, so an inch of his small intestine went without adequate oxygen for a short time, causing his tummy to puff up. Thank God for our neonatologist who caught it early. Thomas required surgery at one week of age to remove the affected part of his small intestine. Only four days after his healthy sister, he came home with an ileostomy—the ends of the intestine are exposed, and the baby eliminates feces into a bag. After only six weeks, he had gained enough weight to merit further surgery to be "reconnected." All went well, or so we thought, until we were packed up to go home and discovered that Thomas had developed a fistula from a torn internal stitch. A third surgery was scheduled to fix it. He responded well, and we were finally able to take him home.

Our baby was now having a normal bowel movement but developed a bleeding diaper rash. The sweet child had already endured so much; it was just awful to see him in continuing pain. All the specialists felt it would just go away. They halfheartedly suggested a dozen different remedies from leaving his diaper off to various salves. Nothing helped. Thomas was in misery. One afternoon in Kroger's, I ran into an ICU nurse from Northside Hospital who had taken care of our daughter. I begged her for advice.

"When all else fails, you go see Dr. Denmark," she said immediately. Being a hospital-based speech therapist, I had heard of her. The next morning my mother and I took Thomas to see her. She told us right off that if he was eliminating feces after every feeding, he was allergic to his formula (a high-priced specialty one). She recommended soy formula and wrote me a prescription for sulfa cream. His little bottom was burned, but he should be well in four days. After three months of watching him suffer, it was just what we needed to hear, and she was totally right.

She also gave me a stern talking-to about structuring my routine—feeding, sleeping, bathing, and basically enjoying my life and babies. She stressed the need for a baby's stomach to empty before filling it again and how important it is not to be seduced into thinking they're hungry just because they are crying. I should give them their last bottles at 10:00 p.m. and put them to bed for the night. At that point I was so exhausted I felt I was falling backwards when I wasn't.

On the schedule she recommended, both babies were sleeping through the night, happy and calm during the day, and always healthy. Thus began my new life! What started off as tiny preemies suddenly blossomed into big fat babies! At nine months Thomas weighs twenty-five pounds and is "off the chart." We laugh that he looks like a miniature linebacker! Alex weighs twenty pounds and is in the 75th percentile.

Dr. Denmark is the grandmother, doctor, and neighbor everyone should have. We take the children back for checkups, and for ten dollars a visit we get counseling as well as sound medical advice! We leave feeling all is right with the world because of her positive attitude toward family, work, and love. She's hilarious. She told me a cow could raise her children better than I do because she doesn't have a brain to confuse her the way I allow mine to do. She told me to think. She stressed that I know what to do and should just go home and do it. That's what makes Dr. Denmark so special. She truly believes in the competence of parents—more so than we do. By empowering us, she knows we'll be better able to care for our children. As she so aptly put it, she can't afford to retire because she has too many parents to whip into shape. I'm grateful to be one of the many to say, "Thank you, Dr. Denmark."

—*Justine Glover*
Cumming, Georgia

Danielle had constant ear infections. By the time she was two, we joked with her doctor that she should get "frequent flyer" status for all the fifty-dollar visits we were making. She was also on the most expensive antibiotic, Ceclor (another fifty dollars a pop) which didn't always work. With one to two infections a month, it was terrible for all of us.

Six months later we moved to Cumming and heard about Dr. Denmark. She told us simply to get her off milk and the infections would stop. Sure enough, she's six now, and there hasn't been another. I ran into her old pediatrician and related this to him. His response was, "She was two years old and that's when kids tend to grow out of them anyway." What a closed mind to the value of proper eating!

—Eric and Tiffany Moen
Suwanee, Georgia

At 12:06 p.m. on April 17, 1993, my only son, Michael Taylor Cromer was born. He was a healthy eight pounds, thirteen ounces and twenty-two inches long. I was told by the hospital nurses always to lay him on his side or back. When we returned to the pediatrician for his two-month check up, he noticed a flat spot on the back of his head. The pediatrician told me to begin to rotate him from side to side and bring him back in a month. If the flat spot had not shaped up, he would send us to a surgeon who would reposition the bones in his head that had grown together. Needless to say, I stood there in total shock. I did not know what to do except pray and cry.

Two friends from church had been trying to get me to go to Dr. Denmark, but I was skeptical because of her age. Well, after I was told what I was told by that pediatrician, I was willing to try anything. So I called my friend at church and asked her to please take me there. Dr. Denmark checked my son out and said that he was perfectly healthy. Naturally, this relieved me of a major burden. She told me not to ever let anyone cut on my child's head. I was to begin placing him on his stomach and as he grew older his head would reshape itself naturally. Today my son is nineteen months old, and you cannot see any sign of the flat spot.

I thank God for Dr. Denmark. She has saved us lots of money and tears. She made me feel I could be a mother without the help of a doctor. I would recommend her to anybody!

—Jenny Cromer
Buford, Georgia

From Afar

Dr. Denmark is the wisest person I've ever known. She told us to change Nicholas' diaper with him lying on his tummy! It works!! It was easier to clean him and we didn't get sprayed. When he was born, the hospital told us to put him on his side to sleep. Other people told us to keep him on his back. Dr. Denmark's advice made the most sense to us. She said to place four bath towels under the crib sheet and keep him on his tummy. We followed Dr. Denmark's advice, and our son had a beautifully shaped head. We never worried that he would suffocate, because the towels gave him enough ventilation, should he sleep face down. He also had great control of his head at an early age because lying on his tummy gave him the ability to turn it from side to side.

We started out with a pediatrician close to home and would see Dr. Denmark (an hour away) from time to time. After just a few visits we realized that her words of wisdom, 65 years of experience, and godly attitude made the long drive worth it! Now when Nicholas is sick, we go straight to Dr. Denmark! She truly loves children; and in my opinion, she is the best doctor in the world. I love her to death!

—Melanie Y. Doris
Fayetteville, Georgia

I grew up on Glenridge Drive near where Dr. Denmark had her office. I now have five children from one month to eight years old. Though we live in Dallas, TX, I have never taken my children to a doctor here. I go back to Atlanta often, and we see Dr. Denmark. We were home this Christmas and took her our newest. After nursing my other four I thought, no big deal. He looks like all the others, so he'll be like they were. But at five weeks, he only weighed eight pounds, thirteen ounces less than at birth. Dr. Denmark said I was starving him and told me how to get him on a schedule, nursing first and then bottle feeding. I now have a baby who sleeps through the night and is perfectly healthy.

I home school my children and treasure the practical advice and love she gives. Because of Dr. Denmark, six-year-old Mary-Elsye wants to be a baby doctor with her office next to Dr. Denmark's. In case there's a question, she can run over and ask her!

We even called her on a ski trip to Colorado when we thought my husband was very ill. The Denmark Milk-of-Magnesia (plus enema) treatment worked wonders. He even shared it with the CEO of his company while they were in New York on business. The man thought he was crazy, but it was that or the emergency room. He chose the treatment and is now a believer. The lives she has touched are many. I thank God so much for her.

—Jan P. Winchester
Copell, Texas

As a missionary living in a foreign country, I have a very special place in my heart for Dr. Denmark and her advice for raising children. I first became acquainted with her after the birth of my first child. We were living in California at the time, but a friend of mine in the Atlanta area told me about the "revolutionary" ideas and concepts that Dr. Denmark had to offer in her book. In an age of "demand feeding and free living," her advice certainly seemed something new. We realized her "plan" was based on Biblical principals and good old-fashioned common sense. We chose to follow her advice, and her book became an invaluable source of information for us. We traveled the United States for a year and a half before coming to the mission field; and *Every Child Should Have a Chance* was a constant companion, helping us to give our daughter the greatest opportunity to learn and grow.

Our second child was born overseas, and we again sought encouragement and advice in the pages of Dr. Denmark's book. We owe her a great deal and praise God that He has allowed us the privilege of knowing such a dedicated and loving person. Thank you, Dr. Denmark, for your influence in our lives and the lives of our children.

—*Pam Campbell*
Argentina

Thank God!

Not once, but twice has Dr. Denmark helped my daughter. The first time was in 1994, when five-year-old Danielle was on antibiotics and inhalers for croup. We spent hundreds of dollars, but after 11 days, she wasn't much better.

I heard Dr. Denmark was still in practice and immediately called her. To put it mildly, not only did she cure my daughter in three days, she told me what was wrong with me during my pregnancy after five obgyn's couldn't diagnose the problem. I had been bed-ridden with Danielle for six months, and was told only various things that were incorrect. I told Dr. Denmark my symptoms, and she said right off, no question about it, I had had placenta previa. She charged me only eight dollars—after we had already spent so much.

The second time she blessed us was this year when Danielle was rushed to Scottish Rite Emergency with fever, rash, croup, and vomiting. We spent 6-1/2 hours in the waiting room, and they wouldn't allow her to eat or drink. At last the pediatrician came in for ten minutes max to tell us the strep test was negative, but they would do another one. He gave her antibiotics for two days and said they'd get back to us. Well, Danielle kept getting worse and finally, after eight calls, they told me the test was again negative. I went immediately to Dr. Denmark and after only ten minutes, found out Danielle had a severe case of scarlet fever! She could have died! I cried my eyes out all the way home, thanking God I'd gotten her to Dr. Denmark just in time.

Danielle was well in three days! Dr. Denmark is an angel. My daughter remains well, and hopefully we will not have to take her tonsils out because of having such a severe case of scarlet fever. She had all the symptoms. If I just had gotten her to Dr. Denmark the first day, she would not have suffered so. When we returned later to Dr.

Denmark for a follow up, she couldn't believe how quickly Danielle had recovered.

"This is a miracle," she said. "These glands aren't even swollen!!" I just cried with joy, hugged her, and thanked her up and down! God bless this lovely lady who really cares for our children.

—*Diane Leonhardt*
Marietta, Georgia

The first time I ever heard Dr. Denmark's name was in 1980 when I was expecting my first child. Friends who were also just starting their families mentioned her while discussing how to choose a pediatrician. I was amazed to hear of the incredible woman who, in her eighties at the time, was still practicing medicine and getting rave reviews from everyone who knew her. I came to find that you don't just "know" Leila Denmark, you "experience" her! I was encouraged on all sides to select this wise doctor. But thinking she certainly wouldn't be around much longer and wanting to be practical, I found a younger physician. Fifteen years later, she's still going strong. By the way, my previous pediatrician quit his practice seven years ago to go into hospital administration!

I probably would never have met Dr. Denmark had it not been for a crisis that struck our family in 1990. It was mid-October when my husband developed a deep and troubling cough. It got progressively worse, but stoic that he is, Brent chose not to see a doctor and just ride it out. A couple of weeks later he and his brother left for a two-week trip to Germany, where the cough grew worse. That same night, almost-two-year-old Abigail began a dry, irritated cough that didn't alarm me at first. As the days went on, it got worse. Soon she was waking up in the middle of the night with spasms that lasted for ten or fifteen minutes and ended with gagging and choking. One afternoon during her nap, my oldest son rushed downstairs to tell me that Abby was choking and turning blue in her crib. I found her as she was recovering from what I later discovered was a seizure. I immediately took her to our family physician, who diagnosed the problem as sinus drainage. Though she had no other indications, he prescribed Tylenol with codeine to help her sleep at night (no lie). Needless to say, I wasn't satisfied but didn't know what else to do. Deciding against the Tylenol "treatment," I chose to wait and see how the next few days went. She had no other symptoms and didn't seem to feel bad or be in any immediate danger. My husband was due home then and could help determine what to do. Her cough continued to worsen considerably, and after another middle-of-the-night spell, I checked our medical books to see what I could find out. I literally went cold at what I read. She probably had whooping cough, a childhood disease especially dangerous for those under two. We also had a newborn son who had started coughing.

Over the years I had heard about Dr. Denmark's work in developing the pertussis vaccine, research that undoubtedly has saved thousands of children from its ravages. If anyone could recognize the disease, it would be Dr. Denmark. I called her office, and much to my surprise she answered her own phone.

"Has she run a fever?" she asked. She hadn't. I was relieved, thinking maybe I was wrong after all.

"Well, she probably has whooping cough. Bring her in immediately," came the shocking reply.

We arrived at her quaint country office, where she ushered us in the back door so as not to infect those in the waiting room. Abby started coughing during the examination. She began to lose her breath, turned blue, and suddenly went limp. Her eyes rolled back in her head and her body began to convulse. I stood with our six other children looking on helplessly and begging Dr. Denmark to do something. It seemed hours before she began to come out of the seizure characteristic of whooping cough. All the while, Dr. Denmark was calm and controlled, talking to Abby and encouraging me at the same time. She quickly confirmed my fears, saying it was a classic case. She wished she could take her to the Medical College of Georgia in

Augusta to teach the students what it looked like. Apparently, there was a tremendous amount of misdiagnosis going on. How well I knew!

After Abby had recovered from the seizure, Dr. Denmark explained why she had spent so long seeking a way to fight pertussis. In one week's time back in the 1940s, she had helplessly watched three children in one family die of the disease that took thousands of lives before the days of vaccines and antibiotics. I was stunned by her story and feared deeply for my little girl. Then three-month-old Josiah started coughing. She asked how long he'd had it.

"Well, if he lives through the week, he'll probably make it," she replied casually, as if predicting a thunderstorm. I was paralyzed with terror at her words, but she gave me a prescription for an antibiotic and detailed instructions on administering it. The drive home is a blank. I do remember imagining preparations to bury my two youngest children.

I called my husband, who had just arrived home the day before. Word traveled fast through our church and circles of friends. They began prayers and started organizing. For the next three weeks we would spend night after night medicating the children every three hours and sitting with them while they coughed out all their air, turned blue, and vomited. As they gasped for breath, we heard the characteristic "whoop" for which the disease is named. I phoned Dr. Denmark every day with my questions and fears.

"I'm so glad you called. How's the baby?" she'd ask. What a blessing to hear her reassuring voice telling me I was doing fine treating them and that it simply took time to get them out of the woods. A lot of naysayers insisted our children should go into the hospital, have respiratory therapy, be on all sorts of medicine, even that I take them to a "real" doctor. Each time a suggestion came, I called Dr. Denmark and in a roundabout way asked what she thought. "Honey, you're listening to your friends again," was her answer. "Just follow my instructions, and don't worry about what others say."

During this time Dr. Denmark's husband was suffering from congestive heart failure, and she was caring for him at home . They had been married for over sixty years, I think, and it must have been agonizing for her to watch him deteriorate before her eyes. Yet she never once made me feel as if my frantic calls were any sort of nuisance. Just the opposite was true. Her compassion poured out upon our family in the midst of what must have been the heaviest trial of her life. He died just as our little ones were beginning to recover. I believe God used her to save the lives of our precious children. We'll be forever grateful for the unselfish and sacrificial way in which she gave herself to our household. There will never be another like her.

—*Laura L. George*
Woodstock, Georgia

Titus 2

Paula Lewis, Windy Echols, and Suzanne Miller, who wrote the following letters, are Titus 2 mentors (see Titus 2:3-5). Their training from Dr. Denmark has played a large part in enabling them to be counselors and a blessing to thousands of young mothers. Paula has also had the time and privilege of seeing her own daughter and granddaughter-in-law become "Denmarkers" too. **(See Paula's daughter's testimony on pages 271-273 and her granddaughter's on pages 269-271.)**

I have such wonderful childhood memories of dear Dr. Denmark. There were four children in our family and each was helped by her through various illnesses. My oldest sister once had a serious case of scarlet fever, and all of us came down with whooping cough— even Mother. Dr. Denmark labeled Mother's illness "the nurse's cough!"

Mother would always pack a lunch when we went to Dr. Denmark's because we never knew how long the wait would be. No one scheduled appointments, so every family waited in line. Dr. Denmark always checked newborns and seriously-ill children first (separately of course). Mother allowed those of us who were well to mingle with other children at the clinic.

Dr. Denmark was the only doctor we went to, and Mother followed her advice to a "T." I remember she always fixed a big, hot breakfast. We were seldom sick and I believe it was because we ate right. My siblings and I are now in our sixties and all still in good health.

When I became a mother, Dr. Denmark was 63. Several family members and friends insisted she was too old and would probably retire soon, but I knew I couldn't do better than take my children to her. She taught me to care for them in every way and loved all of her patients and mothers, especially those who followed her instructions!

I tried to do everything she said to make my children healthy, strong, and sweet. Dr. Denmark always made me feel like I was the best mother she knew. She had confidence in me as a mother, and because of that, I gained confidence and still have confidence today.

Our son adored Dr. Denmark. She actually helped us make an educational decision for him which we believe was pivotal in his success in school and career. He had a late fall birthday, and Dr. Denmark supported our plan to delay first grade until he was seven to give him extra time to mature.

This decision proved to be a wise one. He graduated with honors from high school and went on to do undergraduate and graduate studies at Georgia Tech. Although he and his wife were not able to have their own children, my son often passes child-training tips we learned from Dr. Denmark on to friends. He is always ready to tell other couples how to train newborns to sleep through the night!

Our daughter has been blessed to be the mother of twelve children! Dr. Denmark helped her so much and we have many sweet memories of our visits to her office together, usually for a newborn checkup. My grandchildren learned to love her and listen to her many words of wisdom about how to get along well in this life. They have grown to be healthy, strong, well-disciplined individuals who are willing to work for their aspirations.

I am happy to say that we now have another generation of "Denmarkers"! Our oldest grandson and his wife have been blessed with four beautiful daughters, two of whom are identical twins. These children have never met Dr. Denmark face-to-face, but have benefited from her advice through their grandmother (my daughter), who is a pro at guiding young moms.

Every child does deserve a chance; and it has been my joy to take family and friends to meet and learn from Dr. Denmark. I must say she has been more like a grandmother to me. I believe in the work of her life and wish every mother could have the joy and pleasure God meant for women to experience in their families. I wonder what I and my offspring would be like had I not followed my dear mother and not had the influence of Dr. Denmark in my life. I am truly thankful to God for her.

—*Paula Lewis*
Smyrna, GA

As I sit here looking at a photo of my seven children taken with Dr. Denmark, my heart is warmed and I have to laugh. The laugh is because I remember we forgot to pack a pull-up for my youngest that day…and what we hoped would not happen…HAPPENED when this picture was being taken. Right after the photo, my wonderful husband scooped up the children and took care of the problem, so I could finish my visit with Dr. D. I held her dear, little hand and thanked her once again for everything she had done for me and for sooo many others.

We met Dr. Denmark back in 1988 when I was expecting my first child. Like most newly-pregnant women, I was drawn like a magnet to every baby in sight. I noticed the mothers and observed what kind of experience they were having with their babies. It was significant that some were having a peaceful, enjoyable time while others appeared to be in various stages of miserable exhaustion. My observations led me to greater curiosity after I heard mother after mother say, "Oh! I take my children to Dr. Denmark, the 89-year-old pediatrician. She has a great baby schedule…." Soon I couldn't wait to meet this doctor, although I was a little worried she might pass away before we got the chance!

My husband and I finally met her on a Thursday when her clinic was closed. With only eight weeks to go till my due date, we walked into Dr. Denmark's big, white house and spent two relaxed hours with her, as she calmly and patiently answered all of my childcare questions. We were convinced that hers was the method for us.

By the time my sweet Emily was six months old, mothers were coming up to me to ask baby questions. The summer of 1989, my husband and I were in Colorado for some ministry training, and a group of moms begged me (and my friend Liz May) to do a Dr. Denmark class for them. I called Dr. D and she helped me organize the class material. We sold forty of her books. I didn't realize it at the time, but that summer was the beginning of a long mentoring relationship—Dr. Denmark to me...and me to thousands of mothers.

Over the next eleven years, I birthed six more babies, and each time Dr. D was right there to help. As years went by, the mothering ministry continued. I was able to write many articles, do a radio show, teach classes, and finally produce a training DVD (Well-Fed, Well-Rested Baby, see page 228). All these opportunities were about passing on Dr. D's wonderful training to mothers. I feel so incredibly blessed to have been a part of a living example of Titus 2:3-5...the older women training the younger!! God bless you, Dr. Denmark!!

—*Windy Echols*
Jefferson, GA

Because my first trip to Dr. Denmark's office was when I was three weeks old, I never remember a time when I didn't know and love her. One of my earliest memories is of her warming my undershirt in front of her heater before redressing me after an exam. She was not only instrumental in my development and a blessing throughout my life, but the lives of all seven of my children as well. The last time I visited Dr. Denmark as a patient was for my physical exam as an entrance requirement for nursing school.

From the time my first baby was very young, mothers began contacting me for answers to the age-old question, "How do you get your baby to sleep through the night?" Four years into my journey as a mother, Dr. Denmark physically saved the life of one of my children (see Mark's story below), and she "saved" my life more times than I can count as a mother-of-many by applying her methods that worked so well.

For several years I have taught a group of young mothers at our church focusing on the Titus 2 principles of being keepers of the home and lovers of our husbands and children. What a privilege to include Dr. Denmark's philosophy for the feeding, training, and caring of children. Her practical yet loving techniques create an orderly environment for the well-fed, well-rested baby, as well as for a loving and grace-filled home.

On October 31, 1981, my husband and I were awakened at 5:20 a.m. Our nine-month-old son, Mark, was crying softly. I checked him and found him feverish with a temperature of 105.2 degrees. This was unusual. Mark had never been sick—not even a runny nose. I recollected things I had learned from nursing school. I surmised this was probably one of those high fevers brought on by teething or something else of no serious consequence.

After an alcohol sponge bath, Mark's fever dropped to normal and we put him to bed. The next morning he seemed fine. His temperature was actually sub-normal. I nursed him and began feeding him breakfast "mush." Halfway through the mush he suddenly projectile vomited everything he had eaten across the kitchen.

Extremes in temperature coupled with vomiting was not a good sign. It could indicate some central nervous system involvement. I lay Mark on his back and tried to pull his chin to his chest. It would not bend. I also attempted to pull his knees up to his chest without success. We realized then that our precious baby had spinal meningitis. (See pages 47-48)

It was imperative that Mark get to a hospital immediately so I called Dr. Denmark. Egleston was the choice children's hospital, but at that time it had no emergency room and would not admit patients without a staff physician admitting them. We also were anxious for

Dr. Denmark's counsel. To our dismay, we could not contact her. It was Saturday and she was not answering her phone. As I made preparations to leave, we desperately called all of our friends and asked them to pray that the Lord would bring Dr. Denmark home.

We learned later that God had intervened supernaturally. Dr. Denmark had been standing in line with her husband at a football game and received a strong impression that they needed to go home. She insisted to her husband that they return immediately. It was the first time she'd ever had that impression. She later commented, "I've never had anything like this happen in all my life."

Right before we left to go to another hospital I decided to call her one last time. She had arrived in time to answer the third ring and quickly made arrangements for Mark at Egleston. We reached the hospital just before he began having a seizure.

Initially, the prognosis was grim. His attending physician actually left the hospital that night with no hope. God provided a resident, Dr. Timothy Feltis, who stayed up with Mark and did not leave his bedside even after the attending physician had gone. Dr. Feltis told us, "If you're praying people I would call everyone I know and ask them to pray. This baby's life is in the balance." At 2:00 a.m. Sunday morning, we began calling all of our friends again asking for prayer. After church the next day, Dr. Denmark came to check on his progress.

During the following tenuous days, God used Drs. Feltis and Denmark to provide comfort for us and the excellent care Mark needed to survive. We learned later that Egleston chose to do a symposium on Mark as an example of all the things that can go wrong with a patient who has spinal meningitis. Miraculously, he was healed with no residual effects of the disease. We praise God for His mercy in sparing Mark's life and in using him today for His service. Our family is forever indebted to Drs. Feltis and Denmark for the part they played in saving our son.

—Suzanne Miller
Canton, Georgia

Two by Two

Dr. Denmark has spoken truth every time I have encountered her. Once, after her hundredth birthday, she was examining my baby's nasal passages, trying to determine whether the drainage was clear. "Make him cry," she joked. "Crying clears out the passages...we could tell him about the national debt!" (Pretty sharp for a centenarian.)

My sister-in-law and mother of seven had introduced me to "Dr. D," as she lovingly refers to her. I could use more space than this book would allow writing about our many visits with her and the encouragement she has been to our family, as well as the joy that I have received in sharing her book with others! We were blessed with two sets of twins. Her parenting advice has been the primary tool that God has used to keep our children healthy and their parents sane!

Our first twins were born in 1996 and were nine weeks early. They weighed three pounds, ten ounces, and three pounds, eleven ounces, so had to remain in the hospital NICU for a month, where they received excellent care. They needed to gain some weight, increase lung strength, maintain body heat, and have strong sucks for feeding before journeying home.

During part of their stay in the neonatal unit, the twins had feeding tubes inserted in their noses to ensure sufficient nutrition. My husband noticed that it took four hours for the feeding tubes to empty. This observation confirmed Dr. Denmark's claim that it takes four hours for the stomach to digest milk.

It is ironic that part of our discharge instructions were to feed our infants on demand. My husband's response was, "Thank you for taking such excellent care of our babies, but why would we want to feed them on demand when you have already gotten them on such a good four-hour schedule?"

The sweet nurse's response was, "Well, that's what we've been trained to tell you."

Off we headed for home with our two little miracles, toting neonatal gear which outweighed them by many pounds. As soon as

we arrived, we placed them side by side in the bassinet on their tummies and worked hard to maintain that four-hour schedule.

We did not rush to drop the night time feeding (around 2 a.m.),
but simply pushed it forward a little each night. It was done by allowing babies to fuss a few extra minutes each night before feeding
them. By the time our twins reached their actual due date, the middle
of the night feeding had been eliminated. They did cry sometimes
during the night for the next three weeks, but we did not feed them
in the middle of the night past their due date.

You probably hear that preemies need more frequent feedings
since they were born early and are so tiny, but interrupting their
digestion (remember the feeding tubes?) and making their little bodies work harder is not the answer. Scheduled rest, allowing some lung
exercise (crying), and good, solid feedings every four hours works
wonders for infants. The schedule method brings about benefits for
the whole family a lot sooner—trust me!

I nursed my preemies simultaneously, allowing them to stay on
the breast for about twenty minutes. I never felt that the prematurity
of my twins necessitated their nursing longer than this.

Usually I sat on a pallet on the floor to nurse them with my back
against the sofa. Sometimes, I would position us on the sofa or on a
bed, but never in a chair so as to avoid a dangerous "juggling act."
Whichever baby was the most content after nursing would be placed
on his or her belly for some aerobic time (lifting of neck and shoulders to look around) while the other was fed a few ounces of soy
formula from a bottle. Then baby two would get the supplement.

Later, God gave me another set of twins who were not premature and we put them on a schedule too. We followed the same
methods the second time because they had worked the first time!

I encourage parents of newborns to be diligent in scheduling
during those early days. This is best for babies and it is best for parents. Some may encourage you to be more laid back or have a flip-
flop schedule theoretically to "enjoy bonding time" with your babies
individually. I am not sure I would have been able to smile if I had
done so…Seriously, when would I have showered and brushed my

teeth? Moms, let those sweet hubbies join right in wherever they can and want to. I know mine is such a blessing to our family, and it started back in the NICU when he knew all of the nurses by name before I was even allowed to visit after my emergency delivery.

All four children are doing well, and we thank God for that! He keeps me humble. About the time I think I have things under my control, at least one kid enters a new phase, and I am back on my knees for more instruction. Dr. Denmark is one of those special people who remains with you once you meet her. Not many days pass that something she has taught me doesn't come to mind, whether it pertains to parenting or preparing food. It is a special treat to be able to share what I have learned from her with others.

—*Misti Echols*
Stockbridge, Georgia

I loved having twins. Putting them on a schedule made their infancy a wonderful experience! When they were born, I was living in Indiana so didn't know Dr. Denmark. We learned about scheduling from a homeschooling friend. She had birthed her first baby when her husband was stationed in Germany and the attending German nurses instructed her concerning scheduled feedings. Later, we moved to Atlanta and Dr. Denmark confirmed the system I had learned from my friend.

My fraternal twin boys were born thirteen days early and weighed seven pounds, three ounces, and five pounds, ten ounces. At first they nursed well, but on day six they both refused to nurse on the left side presumably because my left nipple is slightly larger and has a different shape than my right one. This nursing "strike" lasted five days.

It was a very stressful time because I really did not want to have to supplement. I believed in the idea that under normal circumstances God enables mothers to provide sufficient breast milk for their babies. I was also confident in the principle that breasts ordinarily produce as much milk as is required by the baby if the mother is healthy and taking good care of herself by drinking enough and getting adequate rest. So I rented an electric pump and kept working with them.

I'd nurse one on my right side and when the other wouldn't latch on my left side, I tried singing, rocking, walking and even reading Scripture, to calm myself more than anything. I cried and I prayed. This meant that at every feeding one of them was alternately bottle-fed with the milk pumped from the left breast.

Finally, Twin One (the larger baby) latched onto my left breast so I nursed him on this side exclusively for perhaps a week until nursing was stable enough to try Twin Two (the smaller one) on the left. Thankfully, he could now nurse on this side, too. Thereafter, I'd nurse them simultaneously for about ten minutes, burped them, and then put them back on the same breast to finish. At the next feeding, I fed them on the opposite side from which they had nursed previously.

They were worked into a four-hour schedule immediately. Twin One cried at about 3-1/2 hours but I would hold him off until four hours. Twin Two was a sleepy baby so I'd have to wake him up and work with him to wake him up enough to nurse. I'd play with his feet, rub his back, and sometimes even undress him. Twin One was 'chomping down' and ready to burp by the time Twin Two had begun eating. They nursed together in the football hold position with the aid of a nursing pillow. I also changed their diapers after feedings in the same order one after the other and bathed them one right after the other to keep them on the same schedule. After play time, they napped together.

It was wonderful, not much harder than having just one baby, until one caught a cold and was thrown off schedule. The brief time we were off schedule was extremely difficult. I was exhausted having to care for them individually all day long and was hardly able to attend to my three other children, the oldest having just turned seven. It made me wonder how any mother could manage to care for twins by feeding on demand.

Getting them to sleep through the night was more challenging. We separated them into different rooms during this time so one's cry wouldn't wake the other. Not knowing any better, my husband and I mistakenly agreed that he would pick them up when they cried and try to cuddle them back to sleep. This did not work! We did not feed them at night, but picking them up gave them the hope of something more to come and prolonged the process. Twin One didn't sleep through the night regularly until one month old. Twin Two (my sleepy one) slept through at around two weeks.

I was very nervous about their first doctor's visit at 2-1/2 weeks. I wasn't sure they were getting enough milk without supplementing, so I made my husband go with me for moral support in case the doctor yelled at me! As it turned out, I didn't need to worry. Twin One grew from seven pounds, three ounces to seven pounds, seven ounces and by two months up to ten pounds, seven ounces! Twin Two (my small, sleepy baby) flourished by growing from a birth weight of five pounds, ten ounces to six pounds, six ounces at 2-1/2 weeks and was up to nine pounds, seven ounces at two months!

Scheduling twins can be done, and it's well worth it! My advice: Believe it can be done and that your babies will thrive once they're on the schedule, but also find an experienced mom you can call for reassurance when you want to give up. I'm very thankful for the friend who encouraged me!

—*Sharon Joseph*
Alpharetta, Georgia

My twin girls were born at thirty-three weeks. They were in the NICU for about 3-1/2 weeks after birth. When they came home from the hospital they were already on a schedule, eating every four hours. The first night they were at home, both of them slept through the night without the 2:00 am feeding. Throughout the next few weeks they did wake up some nights wanting to be fed. I got up and fed them once during the night for the first one or two weeks. After that, I knew that they had slept through the night without waking up to eat and felt that they were fine to do that, so then if they woke up we let them cry until they went back to sleep. They eventually adjusted to that routine. Even though they were preemies and needed to catch up on their weight, they both thrived on Dr. Denmark's schedule, and were a "normal" weight for their age in just a few months.

Because the twins were in the hospital for the first few weeks and I couldn't be there for every feeding, I pumped breast milk. Initially they were fed through tubes, and then learned how to take bottles. Switching between bottle feeding and breast feeding seemed to confuse them and slow down the process of learning to eat, so they were given my breast milk only through bottles while in the NICU. After they came home, I attempted breast feeding for a while, but because they were already accustomed to taking bottles, it was just too difficult for them to learn something new. I continued to pump breast milk and supplement formula as needed until my supply dwindled to almost nothing when they were six months old. At that time I gave them formula until they were ready to be weaned.

When my twins were three months old, they seemed to be a little dissatisfied with just milk, so I began feeding them pureed baby food. Being preemies, they were somewhat behind developmentally for the first few months and had a hard time adapting to spoon feeding. When it was time for them to eat, I pumped some breast milk, prepared their bottles, bottle- and spoon-fed one baby, bottle and spoon-fed the other baby, cleaned everything up, and then it was almost time to begin the whole process again! I still look back on that time as one of the most challenging experiences with my twins. Looking back, I think it may have been better to wait a little longer before introducing baby food. Eventually though, they got the hang of eating from a spoon, and then I was able to feed them in their high chairs at the same time. That made things much quicker and easier.

We continued to follow Dr. Denmark's feeding plan. When they were about four months old, we fed them three meals per day with formula and baby food, then at seven months weaned them from the formula.

Following a schedule was imperative for me. All of my babies have adapted very well to getting on a schedule, and after the initial adjustment they have been happy and satisfied almost all of the time. As a mother I am busy, but I have gotten adequate sleep at night; and

I have been able to plan my life and responsibilities around my babies' schedule. As I have observed other mothers who have fed on demand around the clock, they seem frazzled, frustrated, sleep deprived, and their babies have been fussy. I am so grateful to have had Dr. Denmark's book, and to have the counsel of other people who have used her methods with great success!

—Rachel Booth
Dallas, Georgia

Mother of Twelve

I am a mother of twelve, who loves to be known as a "Denmarker." My oldest daughter is now twenty-nine and my youngest is five. We also have five grandchildren. My grandmother brought my mother to Dr. Denmark, and my mother brought me. I have taken all my children to Dr. Denmark and my grandchildren are "Denmarkers" too. What a blessing she has been to many generations.

Many have asked me to share with them what I have learned from Dr. Denmark about two challenging subjects: training children to sleep through the night, and potty training. Here are a few things I thought of about sleeping through the night.

Dr. Denmark told my husband and me, with our first baby, to teach her to sleep through the night immediately. She said after the 10:00 feeding, to change her and lay her down in her own room. She said to let her cry and not to pick her up during the night. (I chuckle when I think that she said I could go in and "peek" on her to see if there was a snake in her bed…) Our baby simply had to get her days and nights right.

We began this "training" when she was three days old, after we came home from the hospital. That first night was a challenge. I felt awful when I watched her crying so hard that night, but my husband reassured me, "Don't you remember what Dr. Denmark said. She's just getting her good exercise." We stuck with it and did not get her up. When she fell asleep, she slept for six hours!! I woke her up to feed her the next morning. We continued this each night, and she was sleeping through the night consistently in two weeks.

People said, "You just have a good baby…" Well, after twelve "good babies" and a lot of wisdom from Dr. Denmark, each one of them was trained by two weeks! I never nursed any of my babies in the middle of the night, not once, and they never suffered any health issues due to lack of nourishment. I want to reassure every young mother that the system works.

During the training process, if my newborn slept all night until 5:30 (waking a little bit early and crying) I would say to her, "Sweetheart, you have done very well." Then, I would nurse a little early and stretch the next feeding to 10:00 a.m., to get her right back on the schedule.

Just a note: Keep your infant awake from 6:00-10:00 p.m. as much as possible, to help him sleep well. If they sleep all day, they cannot possibly sleep all night, too. Also, keeping a newborn in a separate room next to mom and dad while training, lowers the stress level.

When our first baby was six-months old, Dr. Denmark told me to start potty training her. I couldn't believe it! I went home and told my husband, and he said, "Everything else she has told us has been wonderful. I think you should try it." So I did.

I put her on a little potty chair three times a day after each meal, and she would sit there from three to five minutes each time. My potty chair had a tray on the front, and I gave her a little book and made it very simple and casual. I "grunted" a few times to encourage her…and in a couple of days, she had a bowel movement! When that happened, we praised her a lot. We continued this routine, and it was amazing how quickly she caught on. Now she had some accidents but was definitely getting the hang of it.

I wouldn't scold her if she did not use the potty but always tried to make it a positive experience. The beauty of starting them on the potty young is that they are not afraid of it. When you wait until two, they are estranged and fearful, and you go through about twelve more months of dirty diapers, time and money!!

Eventually, my babies begin urinating in the toilet, too. (They were so used to sitting there.) If they had an accident, I might say, "Oh no! You are messy now! You should have wet in the potty—now you are all dirty." After an accident, I usually did not change them immediately, so they could feel the consequences of the accident.

When they began urinating in the potty consistently, I would tell them as Dr. Denmark instructed me, "Now you are going to wear panties, like Mommy!" or "Now you can wear briefs, like Daddy!" After that, I took off the diapers and did not use them anymore (I have never used pull-ups).

—*Gina Booth*
Marietta, Georgia

Coming Home

There are many wonderful things I could say about Dr. Denmark, but I'd like to tell you about one incident still very clear in my heart and mind. My two-year-old son was very ill with a fever of 104 degrees one cold, windy night. When I called Dr. Denmark around ten o'clock, she told me to come to her office and she would meet us there. You can't imagine the feeling I had when we came up the hill to her precious little farmhouse-turned-office and saw the waiting light burning brightly for us. All the world seemed dark except that welcoming window. I couldn't help crying with relief at how comforting it felt to be heading to our caring Dr. Denmark. She greeted us in her little robe and slippers, and we gratefully placed our son in her loving arms. In a time when it's sometimes difficult to feel welcome in this world, being at Dr. Denmark's is just about as close to "coming home" as you can get! We love her so!

—*Jodi Zorzi*
Woodstock, Georgia

Epilogue
Pain and the Promise

It had been a brief trip, but Eve was exhausted and painfully distressed, having received some shattering news. She traveled through desolate countryside, indulging dark thoughts. Fierce clouds crackled and poured rain on her windshield. Then all was silent save the swish of water, jerking wipers, and swirl of disquieting images.

An agonized cry gushed out, "But Lord, you promised!"

For the enemy has persecuted my soul...he has made me dwell in dark places, like those who have long been dead.[1] *I will greatly multiply your pain in conception, in painful toil you will bring forth children.*[2]

Eve peered blindly through torrents of rain and finally parked on the side of the road waiting, for a lull in the weather.

Oh Lord, be gracious to me: I have waited for You. Be my strong shoulder every morning. My salvation also in the time of distress.[3]

Finally the deluge slowed. She turned the key in the ignition and eased the car back on the highway.

Although the Lord has given you bread of privation and water of oppression, He your Teacher will no longer hide Himself, but your eyes will behold your Teacher and your ears will hear a word behind you, "This is the way, walk in it," whenever you turn to the right or to the left.[4]

Thankfully, she at least knew how to navigate these roads. Eve turned onto a narrow thoroughfare, carefully avoiding collected pools, trying to corral feverish apprehension and choking grief.

Do not fear, for I am with you; do not anxiously look about you, for I am your God. I will strengthen you, surely I will help you...[5] *Those who sow in tears will reap with joyful shouting. He who goes to and fro weeping, carrying his bag of seed, shall indeed come again with a shout of joy, bringing his sheaves with him.*[6]

At last a familiar road came into view. The sky was still dark, but threads of sunlight and blue sky dared to break through a canopy of mist and overhanging branches. By the time Eve reached their driveway, the rain had slowed to a drizzle. The car had barely turned, when the side door to their house flung open and a little form burst forth, hair streaming, bare feet flying towards her down the drive.

"Can I get in?" Eve opened the passenger door and a dripping Hope jumped in with a brilliant smile and kisses.

Children are a gift of the Lord, the fruit of the womb is a reward...[7] *a joyful mother of children...*[8] *I Myself do establish My covenant with you and with your descendants after you...*[9] *I will pour out my spirit on your offspring and my blessings on your descendants; and they will spring up among the grass like poplars by springs of water. This one will say, 'I am the Lord's'; and that one will call on the name of Jacob; and another will write on his hand, 'Belonging to the Lord.'*[10]

The rain had stopped and the sun smoldered behind clouds, emitting a golden incandescence. "Oh Mommy look!" Eve turned her head and was transfixed. The most glorious double rainbow she had ever seen arched its glowing colors across the sky.

"You know, Mommy, what the most wonderful thing there is?" She extended her arms to embrace the sky. "The most wonderful thing is to be alive!" Hope paused, drank in the view, then danced off to alert the others.

...who have displayed your splendor above the heavens! From the mouths of little ones and nursing babes You have established strength...[11] *Truly, truly, I say to you, he who hears My word, and believes Him who sent Me, has eternal life, and does not come into judgment, but has passed out of death into life.*[12]

Every dark cloud had disappeared. Sunshine glimmered on foliage drenched with tears of rain, soon to dry in the consoling warmth. The storm had passed, leaving a cleansed earth and quieted heart. Comfort dispelled fears with Words, kisses, and glowing hues. All would be most well.

Hope was right—it was glorious to be alive. Her Heavenly Father, had made a promise. The rainbow would soon fade, but the promise would never fail.

Eve hauled luggage out of the trunk and squared her shoulders. There was a lot of work and many challenges ahead, but that was okay.

"There is none like the God of Jeshurun, who rides the heavens to your help, and through the skies in His majesty. The eternal God is a dwelling place, and underneath are the everlasting arms."[13]

She looked up into the expanse of a sapphire sky, a crystalline sea of glass.[14] Suddenly, a welcoming chorus sang out, "She's here! Hey, you finally made it!" Strong arms reached out and took her burdens.

Eve smiled midst her pain. She was...He was her... Home.

References

1. Psalm 143:3
2. Genesis 3:16
3. Isaiah 33:2
4. Isaiah 30:20-21
5. Isaiah 41:10
6. Psalm 126:5-6
7. Psalm 127:3
8. Psalm 113:9b
9. Genesis 9:9
10. Isaiah 44:3b-5a
11. Psalm 8:1b-2a
12. John 5:24
13. Deuteronomy 33:26-27a
14. Exodus 24:10; Ezekiel 10:1; Revelation 4:6

Biographical Sketch
Leila Daughtry Denmark, M.D.

By Steve Bowman

Born in Bulloch County, Georgia, on February 1, 1898, Leila Daughtry grew up on farmland granted to her family by the king of England several generations before her birth. Her grandmother had two daughters, one being Alice Cornelia Hendricks, Leila's mother. At the age of 18 she married Mr. Elerbee Daughtry.

When Leila was born, the third oldest of twelve children, her family lived on a four-hundred-acre farm with an assortment of animals and crops. Their cash crop was cotton. She was six when their home burned. They had to live in a hastily constructed shanty until another, larger house was completed.

Both farm and home were run in a scheduled, orderly manner, without fussing, fighting, or parental bickering. Leila's memories are of harmony, mutual help, and agreeable family relationships. Household workers assisted in child care and other duties. She recalls that the children of the black and white families who worked together on the farm were equally well-behaved.

Her parents taught their children primarily by example. They set standards that she sought to emulate. "You get apples off apple trees," she was fond of saying. "If my mother had raised her voice, I'd have raised mine. If I'd seen my mother smoking, I probably would have, too. But I never saw any of that." The even-tempered Daughtrys practiced genteel manners.

Leila's father was a self-educated, well-read Southern gentleman who was always dressed meticulously. He managed the farm operations without doing any of the manual labor. Elected mayor of Portal, he served in that capacity for thirty-five years. Alice Daughtry died of cancer at the age of forty-five, when their youngest son was only two-and-a-half-years old. Elerbee later remarried.

Leila attended the two-room schoolhouse a couple of miles from home, but she didn't begin until she was eight. Before then, she couldn't walk fast enough to keep up with her older sisters.

The young Leila often pondered what interests she might pursue. Greatly admiring hat makers, who were viewed as artists, she taught herself the craft. Next came sewing lessons and the desire to be a clothing designer. After that, she learned to cook and was certain she would be a dietician.

Leila went to high school in Statesboro at the First District Agricultural and Mechanical School, on the campus of what later became Georgia Southern University, not far from her home in Portal. At Tift College in Forsyth, her classmates called her "Doc," probably because of her interest in anatomy and dissection. (Tift was located in the city of Forsyth, not Forsyth County.)

During her college years Leila read a book on India that detailed the need for medical personnel in that country. She decided to become a missionary doctor to the women of India, where taboos prohibited their being examined by male doctors. A life of medical service out there would suit her just fine. However, a growing interest in a certain young man by the name of John Eustace Denmark changed her plans! They had known each other from childhood, but were never romantically linked. After four years at Tift, she and Eustace became engaged. As she told it: "No one would have me, and no one would have him, so we teamed up!" Deciding to teach school in order to pay her debts before marrying, she gave up the idea of becoming a doctor.

Her first job was in Acworth, northwest of Atlanta. She was to teach science in the local high school. Having grown up in a peaceful, orderly home environment, Leila Daughtry was in no way prepared for the challenges of a public school system.

"Miss Daughtry, you're going to teach the meanest kids on earth," warned the professor who met her at the station. She had no idea what he meant, but soon found out. Some of the boys in her class were better than six feet tall, strong and unruly. At one hundred pounds, she was no match for them: On the first day, she defused a tense situation by requesting the boys' help in setting up and breaking down the classroom. During her nine-month stay she never had any trouble with them; they became her friends.

Realizing she didn't want teaching to be her lifetime occupation, she gave it up after another year in Claxton. At this time Eustace received an appointment to Java, Indonesia, as vice-consul in the city of Soerabaya. He secured her promise to wait for him. The two-year assignment put their marriage plans on hold and allowed the eager Miss Daughtry to set her sights on entering medical school in August. But first, she decided to attend Mercer University in Macon to take the prerequisite physics and chemistry. They told her the courses were so difficult that she might as well not attempt them. She wasn't to be deterred.

When she later applied at the Medical College of Georgia in Augusta, she found all the places were filled; she would have to reapply the following year. She asked them to reconsider their decision. They did so, and allowed her to enter the program. Eustace returned from Java in 1926, and Leila completed her degree two years later.

The year 1928 was a busy one for the young couple. They married in the Baptist Church in Portal, on June 11 at high noon, so all the farmers could attend and then return to the fields. "We married on Monday. I cooked breakfast on Tuesday and started work at Grady Hospital in Atlanta," Dr. Denmark reminisced. She began her internship in the segregated black wards under Dr. Hines Roberts. In August of that year, he asked her to join the staff of Henrietta Egleston Hospital for Children. She became the institution's first intern and admitted its first patient.

During that time, Central Presbyterian Church opened a charity baby clinic. She was one of many physicians who donated time to it every week. Two years later, Leila followed Dr. Roberts to Philadelphia Children's Hospital for six months before returning to Egleston and Central Presbyterian. She would continue her work there for the next fifty-six years.

When Mary, their only child, was born in 1931, they set up a clinic in their home on Highland Avenue so she could both care for the baby and see patients. It was during this time that they joined the Druid Hills Baptist Church, where Dr. Denmark maintained her membership until she passed away. Later they moved to Hudson Drive in the Virginia-Highland neighborhood and lived there until 1949, when they moved again to Glenridge Drive in Sandy Springs. At the time, this was very much in the country. Their fifty-two acres afforded privacy and solace from the crowded city. In 1985, the couple made their final move to Alpharetta.

Her beloved Eustace passed away in 1990 with congestive heart failure. His death was a heavy blow, but she continued on with her practice. Until the age of 104 (2002), she maintained a full work load, seeing patients in a 150-year-old farmhouse next door to her home. Due to failing eyesight, she discontinued examining children, but continued advising parents over the phone.

After a severe case of shingles, Dr. Denmark moved to Athens, Georgia, to live with her daughter, Mary Hutcherson. Her phone counseling continued until the summer of 2010 when she suffered a debilitating stroke. April 1, 2012, she passed away peacefully in her sleep at the age of 114. Dr. Denmark was the longest practicing physician in recorded history and the world's fourth oldest person at the time of her death.

Every Child Should Have a Chance, Dr. Denmark's own book, published in 1971, puts forth her basic philosophy of child rearing and has sold thousands of copies around the world. Numerous articles and documentaries by local and national TV have highlighted her work. More than anything, the multitude of children she has successfully treated give testimony to the usefulness of her life.

History records that Leila Daughtry Denmark's greatest accomplishment was her contribution to the development of the pertussis vaccine, to which she devoted 11 years of research. It reveals much about this remarkable woman that she said, "My greatest accomplishment was getting Eustace as a husband. He's the one who enabled me to practice medicine without thinking of money. He helped get me through medical school and allowed me to continue my work at home while rearing Mary. Without him, I could never have done what I have, helping rich or poor who couldn't otherwise get help. There are none too poor or too rich to take care of their children. They just needed to be shown how," she concluded. Few people have ever come close to Leila Daughtry Denmark in providing a loving, helping hand to so many parents.

Special Services and Studies

- Member of pediatrics staff of Grady Hospital, Atlanta
- Member of staff of Central Presbyterian Church Baby Clinic, Atlanta, 1928 to 1983, devoting one day each week to this charity
- Member of staff, Henrietta Egleston Hospital for Children, Atlanta
- Extensive research in diagnosis, treatment and immunization of whooping cough over a period of 11 years, beginning in 1933. Papers covering these studies were published in *American Journal of Diseases of Children* (a publication of the American Medical Association) in September 1936 and March 1942
- Author of a book on child care, *Every Child Should Have a Chance*, 1971. Second edition, 1977; third edition, 1982. Now in its 13th printing

Memberships and Honors

- American Medical Association
- Medical Association of Georgia
- Georgia Chapter, American Academy of Pediatrics (honorary president)
- Medical Association of Atlanta
- Druid Hills Baptist Church, Atlanta
- Selected as Atlanta's Woman of the Year, 1953
- Received distinguished service citation from Tift College, April 14, 1970, as "a devout humanitarian who has invested her life in pediatric services to all families without respect to economic status, race, or national origin. Devoted humanitarian, doctor par excellence, generous benefactor."
- Honorary degree, doctor of humanities, Tift College, June.4, 1972
- Fisher Award in 1935 for outstanding research in diagnosis, treatment, and immunization of whooping cough
- Distinguished Alumni Award from Georgia Southern College,

Statesboro, January 28, 1978
- Honorary president, Georgia Chapter, American Academy of Pediatrics
- Community Service Award for 1980, sponsored by television station WXIA, Atlanta
- Distinguished Alumni Award from Mercer University, Macon, 1980
- Distinguished Alumni Award from Tift College, Forsyth, 1980
- Book of Golden Deeds Award, Buckhead Exchange Club, Atlanta, April 17, 1981
- Citation from Citizens of Portal at Turpentine Festival, October.16, 1982, jointly with husband, John Eustace Denmark, for outstanding achievement and service
- Medal of Honor from Daughters of the American Revolution, Joseph Habersham chapter, Atlanta, October.20,.1983
- Selected as member of Gracious Ladies of Georgia, Columbus, 1987
- Distinguished Alumni Award from Medical College of Georgia, May 2, 1987
- Honored with husband by Mercer University as life member of President's Club, December 4, 1987
- Shining Light Award, Atlanta Gas Light Company, 1989
- Honorary degree, Doctor of Science, Mercer University, June.2, 1991
- Honorary degree, Doctor of Science, Emory University, May,.2000
- Heroes, Saints, and Legends Award, Wesley Woods, 2000

Appendix I
Immunizations Source Charts

U.S. Produced Vaccines from Aborted Fetal Cell Lines

Disease	Vaccine	Manufacturer	Cell Line (fetal)
Adenovirus		Barr Labs	WI-38
Chickenpox	Varivax	Merck & Co	MRC-5 & WI-38
Diptheria, Tetanus, Pertussis, Polio, HIB	Pentacel	Sanofi Pasteur	MRC-5
Hepatitis A	Havrix	GlaxoSmithKline	MRC-5
Hepatitis A	Vaqa	Merck & Co.	MRC-5
Hepatitis A-B	Twinrix	GlaxoSmithKline	MRC-5
Measles, Mumps, Rubella	MMR II	Merck & Co.	WI-38
Measles, Mumps, Rubella, Chickenpox	ProQuad	Merck & Co.	MRC-5 & WI-38
Rabies	Imovax	Sanofi Pasteur	MRC-5
Shingles	Zostavax	Merck & Co.	MRC-5

U.S. Produced Alternative Vaccines

Disease	Vaccine	Manufacturer	Medium
Diptheria, Tetanus, Pertussis	Daptecel / Adacel	Sanofi Pasteur	Several
Diptheria, Tetanus, Pertussis	Infanrix / Boostrix	GlaxoSmithKline	Several
Diptheria, Tetanus, Pertussis, & Polio	Kinrix	GlaxoSmithKline	Several
Diptheria, Tetanus, Pertusis, Hepatitis B, & Polio	Pediarix	GlaxoSmithKline	Several
Hepatitis B	ENERGIX-B	GlaxoSmithKline	Yeast
Hepatitis B	Recombivax	Merck & Co.	Yeast
Hepatitis & HIB	COMVAX	Merck & Co.	Several
HIB	ActHIB	Sanofi Pasteur	Semi-Synthetic
HIB	Hiberix	GlaxoSmithKline	Semi-Synthetic
HIB	PedavaxHIB	Merck & Co.	Yeast
Polio	IPOL	Sanofi Pasteur	Mondey kidney
Rabies	RabAvert	Novartis	Synthetic

There are currently no U.S. produced alternatives for Adenovirus, Chickenpox, Measles, Mumps, Rubella, Shingles and Hepatitis A. Merck & Co. announced in 2008 that their Mumps and Measles alternatives, Mumpsvax and Attenuvax, will no longer be produced. The new version of the Adenovirus vaccine is currently only approved for use for military personnel.

*http://www.rtl.org/prolife_issues/LifeNotes/VaccinesAbortion_FetalTis sue.html

—*RTL of Michigan, Ed Rivet, page editor.*

Note: Other countries may offer a wider selection of untainted vaccines.

Appendix II
Shall We Watch a Movie?*

Residents of a paper mill town will seldom notice any stench wafting through the air. Many have grown up there—it is home. However, when a visitor arrives, he is likely to exclaim, "Yuck! This place stinks! I wonder how anyone can stand to live here!"

This analogy holds true for movie viewers in America. Most of the films produced by Hollywood and watched by Christians are the moral refuse of a dying culture. They stink but nobody notices; the Church has become desensitized.

There are at least two more reasons why Christians do not notice the "stench." Fallen humanity possesses a schizophrenic tendency to compartmentalize: I practice my religion on Sunday, but Friday... well that's entertainment night. Also, many are quick to reject what they perceive as legalism, only to embrace a liberty which veers into licentiousness, often under the guise of becoming culturally astute or relevant.

It has been said that what people choose for entertainment reflects their deepest hopes and delights. That's a scary thought in light of what our culture chooses to view! When choices are made, we ask the wrong questions and consult the wrong people: If I fast-forward all the bad scenes, will this movie be okay? What's the rating on that one? Did Mr. Jones at church like this one? Honey, if I turn this on, do you think it will scare you? Junior, drive over to Blockbuster and pick out some good ones. (Junior shouldn't dirty his mind looking at the covers, much less what they contain.)

Instead, the questions should be: if Christ were present (and He is), would He approve of what I am watching? Does this film edify my children, energize them for good, improve their preception of life?

I (Madia) am not an expert on film production so have no significant credentials to offer in this discussion on movies, save one: I am the virtual "visitor" to Papermillville. My childhood was largely film-free. The visitor in me wants to exclaim, "Yuck, how can they watch this stuff!"

My brothers and I grew up in a small South Korean town surrounded by mountains. I don't remember our family owning a television during those early years. The mountains were too high to receive AFKN (Armed Forces Korea Network). Korean networks were limited and uninteresting to us kids. We spent our spare time outdoors, climbing trees, caring for animals, hiking, and playing numerous games that Korean children played in those days. We had a wonderful time and often got very dirty. It was post-war Korea. Most of our friends were very poor, but American children today are impoverished in a more tragic way. Their poverty doesn't stem from what they lack, but stems from what they are given.

We missionary kids did not live in a bubble. There was plenty of pain, poverty, and illness around us. However, our parents did shield us from the most horrifying elements of their work when we were very young. I saw TB patients, but never watched them in their last moments as my mother did when she was trying to hold and comfort them. Dad avoided exposing us to much of the heart-rending conditions he witnessed in his travels. When we did see something sad or frightening, it was carefully interpreted for us by my mother, whose words and comfort preserved our sense of security.

Probably among the most chilling sights I remember witnessing as a child were the brightly decorated funeral processions that fluttered their way through the narrow streets up to the mountain graveyards. It was easy to distinguish between the Christian and non-Christian funeral processions. In Christian funerals, the attendees and coffin were dressed in white, hymns were sung, tears shed quietly, bravely. There was hope. Non-Christian processions were always brightly tinseled, accompanied by wailing and rice wine. Drunkenness would dull the pain and help family cope with their loss and the hopelessness.

Speaking of wine—so much of entertainment today functions as the rice wine did for the funeral procession. It affords an escape from reality for those who have no hope and cannot seem to cope with their lives. The entertainment of our days is so often mind and emotion-numbing, an overcharged escape into a world where the immature can pretend to be heroic, beautiful, loved, and admired; where the music dictates to them what to feel, what is significant, what is true, when to laugh, and when to cry. When they awaken from their dream, they find life is dull, meaningless, difficult; and there is no one to interpret it for them. Like the drug addict, when they wake up, all they can think about is when can they dream again. *"When shall I awake? I will seek another drink."*[1]

I am convinced that for believers, entertainment should be recreational in the best sense of the word: re-creational. Are we recreated, rejuvenated, refreshed, and inspired to go about our daily activities with more energy? Feast days during Old Testament times must have provided wonderful recreation for the Israelites. I can imagine the Israeli children particularly enjoyed the Feast of Booths.[2]

When our family goes camping, we are struck afresh at the majesty of our Creator by the beauty of natural surroundings. It is a brief escape from the daily "grind" and affords an opportunity to strengthen familial relationships. We come home tired, but refreshed and relieved to return to the luxuries of convenient showers and washing machines.

There is also something very delightful after a hard week to take a few evening hours off and share a story with the children. That's what a movie is: a powerful presentation of a story, if the craftsmanship is good. Surely there is nothing wrong, per se, with stories. Our Lord used stories to teach. But we should ask ourselves, "Is this the right kind of story, and what effect does it have on me and my family?"

Job made a covenant with his eyes not to lust after a virgin.[3] Shouldn't we make a covenant with ours not to willingly see anything that would sully our minds and hearts? "Does this movie really sharpen my understanding of history or am I enjoying the heady, adrenaline surge brought on by graphic battle scenes? (People got a thrill at the Colosseum, too.) Does this film increase my appreciation for the beauty of relationships or does it foster insatiable desires forbidden by law or providence?"

A well-crafted movie is powerful. According to Geoffrey Botkin, Christian film director, "A movie is a grand collaboration of ten separate artistic disciplines."[4] Its message is usually presented in story form (not propositionally), thereby easily bypassing mental analysis to pierce the heart and emotions on a subconscious level. Such a medium can effectively mold an individual's world view, values, and ethics without the viewer being cognizant of what's happening. By its very nature, artistic or aesthetic workmanship reveals most clearly whom or what one worships. The director is sharing his heart and beckoning to you, "Come, let us worship together."

Hollywood is also money-minded. The market is studied carefully, so that a film will appeal to certain mindsets. *Titanic* obviously appealed to starry-eyed, discontented, adolescent girls. Hollywood made millions off a distorted historical account and probably contributed to the demise of a thousand disgruntled teenage females.

The Bowman household has a general policy: If there is any question about the suitability of the film, it is to be previewed by a few (usually mom and dad) before the family sees it. Recently, one of our sons asked me to preview *Avatar.* It was reputed to have great computer-generated images. He wanted to study it technically, but wasn't sure all the images were appropriate, especially for a young man.

I watched the movie and yes, the special effects were fabulous! I was also amazed at how primitive its message was. The pantheistic spiritism was reminiscent of animism my dad encountered as a rural evangelist in Korea. Many country villages clustered around a "spirit tree," and woe to him who disturbed that tree.

My guess is that the target audience for *Avatar* must have been the hormone-driven adolescent male. Not only would the coarse language appeal to him, but here was his fantasy world where he could return to Eden without facing the flaming sword. He could vicariously "prove himself" by climbing wild terrains, leaping and grappling with ferocious creatures, soaring magnificently through the air to victory, and…of course, there is the sexy, almost-naked, blue creature (blueness minimizes her nakedness so parents won't be shocked). This "lovely creature" picks him as her mate because he is such a hero!

Hollywood made millions, and the American public is now more pantheistic, more pagan, and well, more foolish, because that's what paganism always is — foolish (Isaiah 44:12-20).

The sad thing is that our society desperately needs heroes. Not the phony, mouse-moving, remote-punching, glazed-over variety, but the real kind. We need true heroines who will stop chasing after Greek mirages of perfect body and perfect love and be willing to say like Mary did, *"Behold, the bond-slave of the Lord; be it done to me according to your word."*5 We desperately need true heroes like David who said to his enemy, *"You come to me [with earthly weapons], but I come to you in the name of the Lord of hosts..., and the Lord will deliver you up into my hands."*6 We need heroes who will be openly and unashamedly Christian in all spheres of society, willing to deny themselves and put away childish things for those they love.

If Christians are careful, they can learn technique from master artisans like the incredibly talented men who crafted *Avatar*. I was reminded of Jubal, the son of a crass murderer, who was the inventor of musical instruments.7 Shepherd David plundered Jubal's "technology" and used it to quiet demons and compose Spirit-inspired music.8

Another movie Steve and I previewed was *Dark Knight*. Friends told us it was a great movie for kids: no blood and gore and a clear portrayal of evil. We made one of our few trips to the theatre to see it. Yes, it was definitely a portrayal of evil. But there was a revelling and glorifying of that evil. We saw again and again the Joker's sadistic delight in cruelty. He, not Batman, was the main character. Was it any surprise that the actor died soon after playing this part? It's not healthy to immerse yourself in the role of a demon.

We nixed *Dark Knight* for the family. It would not be an edifying experience. *Dark Knight* didn't meet the qualifications of Philippians 4:8, *"Whatever is true, whatever is honorable...let your mind dwell on these things."* Some of our friends were rather amused at our decision. "What, even your teenage boys can't handle this?" (Incidentally, I've never understood what's so brave about sitting in front of a TV screen). Actually, the most disturbing response was from two nine-year-old boys at a former church. When they found out our guys weren't going to see it, the response was, "What? That's too bad. The Joker is so cool!"

Back to the issue of children—there are two characteristics of children that are salient to this discussion. We all know that children are impressionable. I have often been amazed at how quickly they pick up on nuances, attitudes, and even accents. They are little sponges, especially when it comes to bad behavior. God made little children to be easily influenced so that Christian parents would have an opportunity to teach them the Truth. How can we as parents, in good conscience, set them in front of a powerful movie screen, where they will be taught a humanistic, often Marxist, pantheistic world view. It absolutely doesn't make sense. What could be more of a stumbling block?[9]

The other thing we know about children is that they are vulnerable. They are physically, emotionally, and spiritually more vulnerable than adults, and at an early age they can't always distinguish between reality and fantasy. This vulnerability is coupled with a deep need for security and protection. A sense of security provided early on by parents enables them to mature. As they grow, parents should teach them to find their ultimate security in Christ. Apart from a sense of security, they are stunted in their ability to mature.

Children need to be introduced to the painful realities of life, with careful interpretation, instruction, and comfort at hand. Those who have been exposed prematurely and unaided to violence, pain, or emotionally-charged scenarios will develop coping mechanisms—they have to. They will usually become desensitized or emotionally unstable. We have witnessed this within our own circle of aquaintances. How can traumatized children grow into strong adults? Those who by nature tend to be more sensitive are too busy licking their wounds and protecting themselves to be able to reach out to others. Children less sensitive become calloused and unfeeling. They cannot empathize with others because their hearts are *"covered with fat."*10

This spring we learned to sprout tomato plants from seeds. After sprouts grow a few inches, they are exposed to the outdoors carefully, a few hours at a time, so they will grow to be healthy and strong. When mature and strong enough, the sprouts are planted in the garden to produce beautiful fruit (the analogy is obvious).

I made the mistake—please don't get me wrong; we have made our share of mistakes in this area—of allowing one of our children to view a tense mystery before she was old enough. Years later, she confessed that the experience was frightening. She hardly slept the first night after viewing it. Often children are too dazzled or embarrassed to express their true feelings. They don't want anyone to think they are babyish or immature.

Dr. Leila Denmark, who practiced pediatrics for over 70 years, insisted that one of the major causes for sleep disturbances in children was frightening images on the screen. She recommended that children watch very little television or movies. The few programs they do watch should not be fast-paced, emotionally intense, or frightening. She recommended they watch programs that are "gentle." Gentle doesn't mean insipid, clichéd and sappy. Gentle stories can be simple, true, and deep. These are stories suitable for children. As they grow in maturity, parents must continue to exercise discretion and not get cajoled into making unwise movie decisions. Who is supposed to be guiding whom?

Dr. Denmark grew up in the early part of the last century. Her father was a farmer in South Georgia. During the winter, when there was less to do on the farm, the community would gather for entertainment nights. There would be songs, speeches, and often dramatic poem recitations. This was before the time of radio and television drama.

Dr. Denmark remembered that after a tragic poem was recited, she would sometimes see tears rolling down the cheeks of the weather-beaten farmers. Some of the older ones had fought bravely in the War between the States. They were tough, strong men, but their hearts were not desensitized.

I hope our children will grow into strong, secure, and sensitive adults, sensitive to beauty, pathos, and the needs of others. I want them to be horrified (not afraid) of evil. I want them to be like our High Priest who is touched with the feeling of our infirmities, to be able to weep with those who weep, rejoice with those who rejoice. We pray that the Word of God will be the music of their souls (not theme songs in a film), teaching them when and what to feel, think, and do.

Life is far more fascinating and profound than any movie depiction, if we only had eyes to see it. Maybe if we and our children would stop breathing the soporific stench of Hollywood we would wake up and be able to make really good stories—not coarse, shallow, stupid stories which pervert, distort and sully our hearts, and dull our sensibilities—but really wonderful stories which refresh and sharpen our perspective to better appreciate the richness of life in its tragedy, beauty, humor, complexity and profound relationships. Maybe then, God would give us master craftsmen like Bezalel, the son of Uri, who was *"filled with the Spirit of God, in wisdom, in understanding, and in knowledge, and in all kinds of craftsmanship."*[11]

The King is sitting at His table. May that same mysterious Spirit blow over the gardens of our lives, recreating, releasing, wafting the aroma of Mary's spikenard, spices, and choice fruits unto Him whose love is far better than any wine.[12]

This article was written for an online church discussion group.

References

1. Proverbs 23:33-35.
2. Leviticus 23:34-44.
3. Job 31:1.
4. Geoffrey Botkin, Hollywood vs. Christian Culture (Vision Forum Ministries CD, 2005).
5. Luke 1:38.
6. 1 Samuel 17:45-46a.
7. Genesis 4:19-24.
8. 1 Samuel 16:14-23, Psalms.
9. Matthew 18:6
10. Psalm 119:70
11. Exodus 31:2-3.
12. John 12:1-8, Song of Solomon 1:12, Song of Sol. 4:13-16, Song of Sol. 1:2, 4b.

Appendix III
Bowmom's Maxims

Parenting can bring enormous fulfillment and joy. But, Moms, do you ever feel like you're in a battle? There are battles with the laundry, the dishes...and the sinful attitudes (both ours and the children's!) Sharpening and shooting our *"arrows"*[1] can be tough. I take comfort in the following verse: *"He trains my hands for battle, so that my arms can bend a bow of bronze."*[2]

If our great enemy, Satan, cannot lure us into flagrant sin, his next tactic is to distract us from what's most important. Life is full of distractions. It always helps me to focus if I periodically write down my goals and maxims.

The following are my personal lists of battle maxims developed through the years. Please understand these represent mothering techniques which I haven't fully mastered. This "Bowmom" is still learning, and I haven't shot all of my arrows. Hopefully, reading these maxims will inspire you to write your own.

Relational
1. Nurture relationships with Christ through prayer, Bible study, family worship, and church.
2. Remember we live in a corrupt society, and God calls us to holiness (separateness).
3. Train soldiers for Christ's kingdom.
4. Model submission and respect for authority.
5. Focus on heart attitudes (what are their motivations?).
6. Require quick, cheerful obedience.
7. Be consistent.

8. Home educate.
9. Set up clearly defined family policies based on Scriptural principles.
10. In making decisions, don't give in to the wrong kind of pressure. Look to principles, not child's desires, as guidelines. (We want to honor Christ, not satisfy whims.).
11. Take time to talk.
12. Be a good listener and seize mentoring opportunities.
13. Pray together about problems, concerns, and anxieties.
14. Encourage mutual kindness and respect.
15. Insist on wholesome social settings.
16. Severely limit time with peers; have lots of wholesome recreation as a family.
17. Carefully monitor TV, video, cell phone and Internet usage as well as the quality of reading materials.
18. Insist on wholesome, good-quality music. Music has a powerful effect on atmosphere and attitudes.
19. Encourage siblings to be best friends.
20. Nurture masculinity and femininity.
21. Be willing to ask forgiveness; make it a habit.
22. Don't make mountains out of mole hills (especially when stressed).
23. Recognize creational differences among children.
24. Try not to humiliate; build up.
25. Balance gentleness with absolute firmness ("akimbo").
26. Be affectionate and make a habit of thanking children whenever you can.
27. As children mature, transition gradually from queen to coach.
28. Look for and nurture signs of the Holy Spirit's working (fan the flame with encouragement and praise).
29. Use trials and conflicts as opportunities to learn and teach.
30. Openly praise, encourage, and admire where appropriate.
31. Pray, pray, pray; forgive, forgive, forgive.
32. Trust Him to bring fruit from labors, and be happy.

Practical

1. Begin each day with the Word and prayer.
2. Slow down (for type A personalities).
3. Occasionally take time out to plan and prioritize.
     Note: Solicit the help of a trustworthy babysitter, if possible, when you are planning and prioritizing. While she corrals the little ones, you can think!
4. Maintain a good, realistic schedule under the direction of your husband.
5. Minimize outside activities; learn to say no graciously.
6. Eat right and get enough sleep.
7. Simplify and streamline (K.I.S.S.- "keep it simple, stupid").
8. "Dejunk" your life (possessions, time commitments).
9. Take time to train and delegate duties (Exodus 18).
10. Set up daily, weekly, and monthly chores.
     Note: Larger families do need more delegation and regimentation, but even with small households, delegating and designating chores take stress off mom and helps develop discipline.
11. Stress diligence, teamwork, and service.
12. Don't expect perfection.
13. Provide accountability where needful and possible.
14. Keep primary workspace picked up (for me it's the kitchen and den).
15. Wear comfortable shoes or slippers while you work.
16. Avoid outside, part-time work for children; encourage home business.
17. Severely limit TV, time on the Internet, and time on the phone for everyone.
18. No video games.
19. Consolidate trips.
20. Learn to work incrementally on big projects (such as writing books!).
21. Don't allow your numerous responsibilities to paralyze you. Simply go on and **do the next thing.**
22. Try to schedule most important things for the morning.
23. Always consider practical implications before agreeing to outside commitments.

24. Unless you are a high-energy person, seldom agree to last-minute changes in plans.
25. When God brings interruptions into your life which disrupt your schedule, go with the flow and use interruptions as learning opportunities for all.
    Note: Some interruptions are especially challenging, such as severe pregnancy nausea, extended illness, or tragedy. At times like these, switch to "survival mode." Delegate as much as possible and pare down to bare essentials; i.e., prayer, nourishment, safety for the children, and clean bathrooms.
26. Don't get derailed by providential interruptions. After they are over, get back on schedule.
27. Double up on cooking (cook at least two meals worth at a time).
28. Every mother must multi-task, but don't drive yourself crazy by too much multi-tasking. There's something to be said for finishing one small task before going on to another.
29. Don't attempt projects that require extended, focused attention while babies are awake.
30. Be creative in problem solving (ask God for ideas).
31. When facing an overwhelming task, divide it into manageable moments (even kitchen cleanup can be approached this way: clear glasses first, next dinner plates, and so on).
32. Discover some kind of wholesome, rejuvenating diversion and escape into it occasionally if you can. For some women it might be sewing, for others taking walks, gardening, or reading excellent literature. (This refreshment is especially important for type A personalities.)
33. When you are knocked down, don't give up. Admit failures, ask God for help, pick yourself up and go on.
34. Be thankful at the end of the day for what has been accomplished (even if it seems minimal).
35. Delight in your family!

References

1. Psalm 127:4.
2. Psalm 18:34.

Index

A

Abdominal pain (see Somachache)
Allergies, 11, 12-14, 19, 27-28, 29, 53-54, 90, 110, 243-244, 248-249
    Chapter 8
  eczema, 11, 29-30, 57
  poison ivy or poison oak, 58-59, 133
  rashes, 27-28, 29, 58-59, 110, 113-116
Ampicillin, Chapter 7
Anemia, 21, 36-37, 154-156, 160-161
Antibiotics, Chapter 7
Appendicitis, 48-49
Argyrol, 125
Asthma, 91-92, 114-116, 248-249
Aspirin, 119-120
  dosages, 120
  Reye's syndrome, 72-73, 102-103
Athlete's foot, 60
Auralgan, 125-126

B

Baby food (commercial and home-made), 29-37
Bathing baby, 23-24
Bed-wetting, 159, 272-273
Bee stings, 63
Benadryl, 121
Bites, 63-65
Bleach, 127
Blisters (friction), 62
  chicken pox, 100-103
  poison ivy, 58-59
  diaper rash, 27-28
  burns, 56, 61, 132
  insect bites, 63-64
Blow to head, 65

Boils, 61-62
Broth, 79
Breastfeeding, 8-10, 247-248
Burns (see Sunburn), 56, 132

C

Caladryl, 121
Calamine, 121
Chapped skin, 62
Chicken pox, 100-103
Chlor-Trimeton, 121
Clothing, 24-26, 203-205
Congestion (see Colds), 19-20, 89-90
Conjunctivitis, 66
Constipation, 71-72, 123
Colds, 89-92
Colic, 4-5, 11, 12-14, 16, 242-243, 246
Coughing, 91, 103-104
Cough medicine, 91
Croup, 91-92
Crying, 6-8, 88-89, 241-242, 246-248, 251, 271-272
Cuts, 54
Cystic fibrosis, 104

D

Dairy products, 96, 114, 160-161, 242-244, 249, 252
Dehydration, 72-79
Diaper rash, 27-28, 250-251
Diarrhea, 11, 71-75, 80
Down's syndrome, 8, 17, 98-99
Dramamine, 122
Drinks, 34-37, 158-159

E

Ear infection, 16-17, 19, 94-96, 252
    tubes, 16-17, 95-96, 243-246, 249, 252
Eczema, 11, 29, 57
Emergencies, Chapter. 2, 52, 56, 63, 64, 65, 67, 117
Enemas, 71-78, 122-123, 254
    retention enema (tea enema), 75-76
    standard enema, 73-75
Erythromycin, Chapter 7
Exercise, 177-178
Eye infection, 66, 70

F

Fainting, 67
Feeding
    newborns, 4-15
    three months, 28-32
    four months, 32-34
    five months, 34-37
    two years, 39-41
Feet and shoes, 26-27, 60
Fever, Chapter 5
    emergency, 47-48
Five month infant, 34-38
Flu, 92-93
Flu shots, 93, 238
Formula (see Supplements)
Four month infant, 32-34

G

German measles, 100

H

Headaches, 53-54
Humidifiers and vaporizers, 90-92, 114-115, 248

I

Immunizations, 43-45, Chapter 13, Appendix I
Infectious diseases, Chapter 6
Impetigo, 60-61
Intestinal disorders, 51-53, Chapter 4

J

Jaundice, 21
Jellyfish stings, 59

K

Kenalog cream, 126
Kwell, 123

L

Lice, 65
Listerine, 123

M

Macrodantin, 126
Meningitis, 47-48, 83, 263-264
Menstrual pain, 67

Mercurochrome, 123

Merthiolate, 123

Milk of Magnesia, 124

Motion sickness, 53

Mouth sores, 67

Mycostatin suspension, 126

Mycostatin topical powder, 126

N

Naptime, 20, 34, 37-38, 40
    napping schedules, 42
Needs of children, Chapter.12
Newborns, 4-28
    crying, 6-8, 88-89, 241-242, 246-248, 251, 271-272
    furniture use, 19
    jaundice, 21
    schedules, 4-5
    sunshine, 20
    positioning, 16-19, 233-234, 252-253
    postpartum, 15-16
    weight gain, 15
Nose bleeds, 69
Nursing care, 78-79, 85-86, 105-106, 178-179
Nutrition, Chapter 11
    calcium, 161
    dairy products, 96, 114, 160-161, 242-244, 249, 252
    drinks, 34-37, 158-159
    fats, 161
    fruit, 156-157
    infant (see Feeding)
    mealtime, 162-164
    protein, 154-155
    recipes, 165-173
    sample menus, 164-165
    starches, 156
    sweets, 157-158
    vegetables, 156
Nystatin suspension, 126
Nystatin topical powder, 126

P

Pacifiers, 21-22

Pedialyte, 77, 124

Penicillin, Chapter 7
Petroleum jelly, 125
Premature Infant, 9-10, 30, 250-251, 265-267, 269-271
Pneumonia, 93-94
Pinworms, 40-41, 69-70
Poison ivy or poison oak,58-59, 133
Positioning of newborns, 16-19, 233-234, 252-253
Postpartum, 15-16
Potty Training, 159, 272-273

R

Rashes (general), 58
    diaper rash, 27-28, 250-251
    German measles, 100
    poison ivy or poison oak, 58-59, 133
    scarlet fever, 99, 255-256
    chicken pox, 100-103
Reye's syndrome, 72-73, 102-103
Ringworm, 60

S

Scarlet fever, 99, 255-256
Schedules
    baby schedule summary chart, 42
    newborns, 4-5
    three months, 28-29
    four months, 32-34
    five months, 34-36
    two years, 39-40
    family routine, 174-177, 247-248
Scrapes, 54-55
Scratches, 54
Shingles, 101
S.I.D.S., 17, 232-234
Silvadene cream, 126
Sinus infection, 90, 94
Sleep, 37-38, 175-177
    requirements, 176
    disturbances, 16-19, 20, 40-41, 69-70, 296-297
Smallpox, 101
Spitting up, 4-5, 11, 12-14, 16, 242-243, 246
Styes, 70

Stings, 63-64
    jellyfish, 59
Stomachache, 48-49, 51-53, 71-72
        menstrual pain, 67
        swallowing objects, 48-49, 65
        emergency, 48-49
Strep throat, 96-99
Sudden Infant Death Syndrome (see S.I.D.S.)
Sunburn, 61
Sunscreen, 61, 177
Sunshine, 20-21, 177
Supplements, 7, 10-12
Swaddling, 18
Swallowing objects, 48-49, 65
Swimmer's ear, 68

T

Teething, 28
Thermometers, 124-125
Three-month infant, 28-32
Throat Infection, 96-99
Thrush, 8, 21-22
Ticks, 63
Tonsils, 98-99
Twins, 250-251, 265-271
Two-year-old, 39-41

U

Urinary tract infections, 103, 158-159, 248

V

Vaccinations (see Immunizations)
Vaporizers (see Humidifiers)
Vaseline, 125
Vermox, 127
Vomiting, Chapter 4

W

Weaning, 37
Wheezing, 91-92, 248
Whooping cough, 43-44, 103-104, 109, 256-259
        development of vaccine, Chapter 13
Witch hazel, 125